Eat for Life Diet

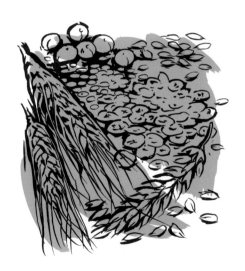

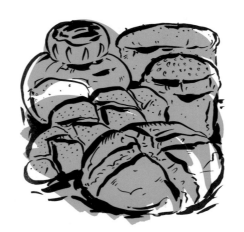

Eat for Life Diet

-

A revolutionary new eating plan

based on the findings of the

World Health Organisation

-

JANETTE MARSHALL AND ANNE HEUGHAN

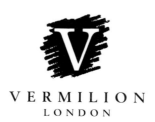

VERMILION

LONDON

Published in 1992 by VERMILION
an imprint of Ebury Press
Random Century House
20 Vauxhall Bridge Road
London SW1V 2SA

EDITORS: Alison Wormleighton and Barbara Croxford
DESIGNER: Terry Jeavons
ILLUSTRATIONS: Ivan Hissey

Printed and bound in Great Britain by Butler and Tanner Ltd, Frome and London.

Contents

Foreword by Professor Philip James

By changing what we eat, and taking regular exercise, we can substantially reduce our risk of heart disease and diet-related cancers. But for most people the most persuasive benefit of a change in diet and lifestyle is losing weight.

I spent five years as chairman of the World Health Organisation committee that published the report *Diet, nutrition and the prevention of chronic diseases*. During this time it became evident that there was a clear way to deal with weight control and the major, diet-related health problems of our times. The same diet that helps prevent heart disease can also be beneficial for avoiding coronary heart disease, diet-related cancers, dental decay, arthritis, osteoporosis — and weight control.

That world scientists have now arrived at this consensus is remarkable when considering that a body such as the WHO has to be conservative. It would be wrong to have ever-changing policies, but the evidence on diet was now not only strong but also longstanding, so a new policy on healthy eating was warranted. New evidence, however, is required to deal with the many unresolved issues.

We were able to recommend a set of nutritional goals which can encompass many different diets. Producing such a document is, however, of little relevance to improving Britain's poor record of diet-related disease and substantial increase in obesity, unless ordinary people are approached directly with the information, in an understandable form, needed to help them change their eating habits.

Motivating people to change is vital if we are going to improve our poor health record. It's estimated that one third of people in the UK are overweight. And if you consider that throughout your entire adult life you should not weigh more than what your weight was at the age of 25, then we have a real problem. As many as a quarter of us are already overweight by the age of 25, and thereafter most people gain more weight.

Overweight people are more likely to suffer coronary heart disease, high blood pressure, strokes, the commonest forms of diabetes, and diet-related cancers, such as breast cancer and cancer of the colon. Disability from hernia, arthritis and gallstones are also far commoner in the overweight. If we can help people to lose weight and preferably to prevent weight gain in adult life then we will go a long was to reducing the burden of ill health in Britain.

I welcome the publication of Eat For Life Diet, which tackles the health problems head on. We need to prevent weight gain but also the many complications which arise from eating an inappropriate diet.

PROFESSOR PHILIP JAMES, MA, DSC, FRCP, FRCP(E), FRSE
Director, Rowett Research Institute, Aberdeen, October 1991.

Food
Glorious
Food

Eat For Life Diet is your blueprint for healthy eating for the 1990s – and beyond. It explains how to make the best choice of good, fresh food and provides recipes so you can cook it to produce delicious dishes. In order to explain which foods to choose, why they are good for healthy eating and slimming and how many, or how much of each to eat, Eat for Life Diet also goes into nutritional details. However, when we talk about fats, starches, complex carbohydrates, fibre, and so on, what we are really talking about is good food. So after reading the Eat for Life Diet story we hope you, your family and friends, will forget all about 'nutrition' and 'calories' and just eat and enjoy in a new and enlightened way.

JANETTE MARSHALL AND ANNE HEUGHAN

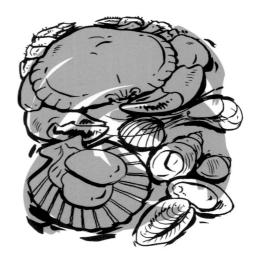

Introduction to Eat for Life Diet

Eat for Life Diet is two things. First, the Healthiest Diet in the World, and second, a revolutionary slimming diet that will help you stay slim and healthy for a lifetime.

Not since the *F-Plan Diet* has there been such a revolution in the way we eat. Like Moses with his tablets of stone, the world's leading scientists have now come down from the mountain top and, with one voice, are giving us a very clear and simple message that will enable us to take the biggest step forward in healthy eating and slimming for the last 20 years.

The message is clear and simple. The healthiest people in the world follow three simple rules which we have encapsulated in Eat For Life Diet. They eat:

1   About half their food as starchy food such as bread, pasta, rice or potatoes.
2   At least five portions of fruit and vegetables a day.
3   A minimum of saturated fat.

These three characteristics are the cornerstone of Eat For Life Diet, both for the slimming plan and for the long term programme for healthy eating.

This revolutionary new approach is based on sound scientific findings – from the World Health Organisation's (WHO) latest report *Diet, nutrition and the prevention of chronic diseases* and the British government's *Dietary Reference Values for Food Energy and Nutrients for the United Kingdom* – making it both safe and effective.

Eat For Life Diet has taken the scientific findings from these reports (and many that have gone before) and translated them into:

- an Everyday Eating Plan
- a 28-day Slimming Plan
- an Easy Option Slimming Plan for busy people.

All are suitable for men and women, and each quashes the myth that bread and potatoes, pasta, rice and other wholegrain, starchy foods are fattening.

~ *The perfect slimming diet* ~

You can start straight away on Eat for Life Diet and it won't be long before you discover that this new healthy eating diet is also the perfect slimming diet. You can stay on it safely for as long as you like. There are no gimmicks with Eat for Life Diet. The foods are low-fat, simple, delicious and as varied – or as ordinary – as you want them to be. You won't be asked to eat grapefruit, or anything else you don't like, ad nauseum. And you won't go hungry.

Just one way of eating, encapsulated in Eat for Life Diet, not only helps protect you and your family against heart disease, diet-related cancers and other less serious health problems, but also helps you achieve your ideal weight.

Unlike very low-calorie diets and crash diets that have gone before, the Eat for Life Slimming Plan is based on a realistic 1,200 calories a day. This in itself reflects the latest thinking on dieting that shows:

- You are more likely to stick to a diet that allows you 1,200 calories, therefore you are more likely to succeed.
- You will find it more filling, satisfying and pleasant to follow.
- While your weight loss will be marginally slower, it will be more permanent.

Twelve hundred calories a day might be commercial poison to the 400 calorie, 800 calorie or 1,000-calories-a-day diet brigade who want you to lose weight quickly so you can put it all back on again and buy their next wonder diet. But if you seriously want to be permanently slim the Eat for Life Diet is the best (and healthiest) way to do it.

Assuming your body uses 2,000 calories a day at present, after a week on the Eat for Life Slimming Plan you will have lost 5,600 calories, the equivalent of 0.7 kg (1^1/2 lb) of fat. With the usual water loss that occurs during the first week of a diet that could amount to as much as a 3 kg (6^1/2 lb) weight loss. After that you can expect to lose a further 0.7 kg (1^1/2 lb) of fat a week – or more if you follow our exercise advice (see page 92). In 28 days you could lose about 5-6 kg (11 lb-1 stone). This is not crash dieting. Weight loss at a such moderate speed is permanent, provided you adopt Eat for Life Diet's lifestyle. Achieving this weight loss on 1,200 calories a day is the least painful way to do it.

Controlling the calories will enable you to lose weight, but to look and feel even better you will need to improve your muscle tone and general level of fitness through exercise. Whatever age you are, it's never too late to start, especially as the latest advice from the Royal College of Physicians is to begin exercise early in life and continue it through middle-age and into old age as a regular part of weight control and keeping healthy.

~ *The Healthiest Diet in the World* ~

Once you have reached your target weight, Eat for Life Diet doesn't leave you high and dry because the other revolutionary aspect of losing weight with this slimming plan is that it stems from The Healthiest Diet in the World (Chapter Two). So after your slimming diet – or if you don't need to diet – just follow the Everyday 2,000 calorie Eating Plan in Chapter Seven which shows you how to put the Eat for Life principles of healthy eating into action.

Adopting Eat for Life's eating plans is not a list of don'ts. It is one of the most positive things you can do for yourself. And combined with other lifestyle changes such as not smoking and taking more exercise, there has never been a better time to do it. Never before have we had such an array of fruit and vegetables in our shops. Eat for Life Diet shows you how to make the most of these, from the everyday to the exotic. Once you have absorbed the principles you can go as mad as you like, experimenting with everything from aubergine to zucchini [courgettes]!

By eating more fruit and vegetables, and starchy fibre-rich foods – the first two recommended dietary goals – Eat for Life Diet automatically achieves the third main goal, reducing the saturated fat in your diet. This should help to save lives lost prematurely to the two scourges of modern living: heart disease and cancer. And cutting down on fat automatically helps you lose weight.

The special health benefits of the Eat for Life Diet come from the newly discovered relevance of Superfoods (Chapter Three). Their built-in nutrient density is yet another of Eat for Life Diet's unique features. You could say it is one of Eat for Life Diet's 'ACE' cards, because the latest scientific evidence suggests eating food rich in vitamins A, C and E (ACE Eating, Chapter Four) will also help protect your health.

With its emphasis on starchy foods (complex carbohydrates or 'CC foods' for short) as opposed to animal products, Eat for Life Diet will revolutionise meal planning and the way you shop. Instead of first thinking which meat or fish to have for your main meal, with Eat for Life Diet your first thought is 'Which starchy food will I build my meal around?' You might choose bread or potatoes, rice, pasta or pulses. Whichever it is, turn to the recipe section which is organised according to starchy food categories, and away you go. Incidentally, just because you 'Think CC Foods First', it doesn't mean you have to become a vegetarian. Many of the recipes contain meat or fish — and there are vegetarian recipes, too.

~ Start now ~

To be your ideal weight and eat the healthiest diet known, choose the whichever Eat for Life eating plan suits your needs.

- If you have some weight to lose go directly to the 28-Day Slimming Plan (pages 65–74), or its Easy Option Slimming Plan (pages 75–80).
- If you want to look and feel your best without slimming as your main priority, turn straight to The Healthiest Diet in the World (page 13).
- Use the uniquely arranged recipe section — classified by CC Food (page 97) — to revolutionise your eating and shopping habits.

F

The Healthiest Diet in the World

or many people, the main attraction of Eat for Life Diet is the fact that it shows us how to eat all we want without getting fat. But in fact it can can also help protect against many diseases, including heart disease and diet-related cancer. In Britain – which leads the world in heart disease – this has to be good news.

~ Adding CCs to our lives ~

Since worldwide scientific research has now confirmed the relationship between diet and disease, we can say with certainty that to feel and look our best we need make only a couple of fundamental changes to the way we eat. We must:

- Ensure that CC foods (complex carbohydrates) – starchy, fibrous foods such as bread, pasta, potatoes, cereals contribute about half our daily calorie intake.
- Eat at least five portions of fruit and vegetables a day.

Altering the diet in this way will automatically reduce the amount of saturated fat we eat without our having to do anything further.

Eat for Life Diet shows exactly how to make these changes, not only as the basis of a 28-day slimming programme, but also as the foundation of a lifetime of healthy eating.

Never before have we had such remarkably consistent advice from scientists about exactly how to achieve The Healthiest Diet in the World. What's more, it seems that just one way of eating protects against a broad spectrum of diet-related health problems. So it's not necessary to select one special diet in order to prevent one particular disease and by so doing put yourself at risk of another disease.

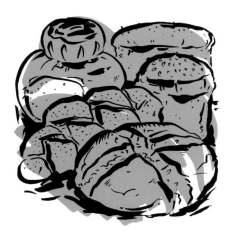

All over the world the people least likely to suffer heart disease, high blood pressure and certain cancers, diverticular disease, appendicitis, haemorrhoids and constipation, are those whose diets are rich in plant food – in other words, starchy CC foods, and fruit and vegetables. Whether this is due to substances in the plants, or the fact that such diets are usually low in saturated fats and animal protein, is not known exactly. It's probably a combination of both.

~ Universal Dietary Goals ~

The Eat for Life Diet is not just another vague exhortation to eat more high-fibre food and less sugar and fat. Instead, it provides practical guidelines for what to eat and how much, based on the latest scientific findings. Scientists are now so confident about their message that they have set universal, or 'population', goals for how much of each type of food we should eat. In particular, upper and lower limits have been set by the World Health Organisation (WHO) for the amount and type of fat, protein, complex carbohydrate and free sugar that should be eaten to be slim, fit and healthy. The British government's recommendations are broadly similar and are given in Appendix 1.

~ Population Nutrient goals ~

Nutrients are expressed as percentage of daily energy/ calorie intake or in grams per day.

	Lower limit	Upper limit
Total fat	15%	**30%**
Saturated	0	**10%**
Polyunsaturated	**3%**	**7%**
Dietary cholesterol	0mg/day	300mg/day
Total carbohydrate	**55%**	75%
Complex carbohydrates	**50%**	70%
Total dietary fibre	**27g/day**	40g/day
Free sugars	0	**10%**
Salt	not defined	**6g/day**

★ *Diet, nutrition and the prevention of chronic diseases*, World Health Organisation, 1990.

Figures in bold are the ones that as a nation we should try to achieve.

The upper limits are the most important figures relating to fats, sugars and salt. In Britain we regularly eat more than these amounts so we need to make sure that in the long-term we eat less fat, sugar and salt. For complex carbohydrates and fibre the lower limits are the most relevant, as these are the most achievable in the West. The upper figures in these categories are more relevant for the people of developing countries, whose traditional diets supply more of these foods than in the West.

The lower limit for polyunsaturates is also important. These fats have to be eaten, as they are essential for health and the body cannot make them.

The zero ratings for saturated fat, dietary cholesterol and free sugars indicate that these foods are not necessary for health. This is not to say that they cannot be eaten ever again, but simply that we should be careful about how much and how often they are eaten.

The British government's new Dietary Reference Values are very similar to the WHO advice for fibre and polyunsaturated fats. They differ a little, however, on saturated fat, total fat and free sugars; some would say they are less draconian. Nevertheless, WHO and the British government are unanimous on the big Eat for Life Diet message, which is to eat more CC foods, fruit and vegetables and to eat less fat and free sugars. If you want to read about the British Dietary Reference Values in more detail, see Appendix 1.

~ What it means in terms of real food ~

The WHO table shown on page 14 means that we should:
• **Eat more bread, cereals, pasta, rice and so on**, so that about half the diet is made up of those foods.
• **Eat more fruit and vegetables**. Aim for 400 g (14 oz) a day, including at least 30 g (1 oz) of pulses, nuts or seeds, which are particularly important for vegetarians.
• **Change the basis of meals**. Instead of meat and two veg, the everyday norm for main meals should now be bread, potatoes, rice or pasta and two veg, plus a little lean meat or fish. In fact bread should accompany every meal, as it does in Mediterranean countries – preferably without butter or margarine. Fruit or a low fat yogurt replaces the sticky pudding.
• **Eat less sugar** because free sugars are not beneficial for slimming

or healthy eating. No more than 10 per cent of calories should come from sugar, whether it's stirred into drinks, sprinkled on cereal or already in sweets, cakes and other manufactured foods.
• **Eat less fat**, especially saturated animal fats. Making the above changes will shift the emphasis away from fatty foods.

~ *Staff of life* ~

Bread has been called the staff of life and for good reason. Bread, potatoes and cereals are low in fat, and bread and cereals are rich in B vitamins, minerals and trace elements. Wholemeal breads and cereals are especially rich in fibre and essential fatty acids.

Contrary to popular belief, starchy foods are not fattening; it's the fat you add that makes them high-calorie. That's why Eat for Life Diet opts for boiling or steaming potatoes, rice, couscous, bulghur wheat, buckwheat, pasta and noodles rather than frying them. Where frying is used, it is done quickly and with the minimum of oil, as in stir-frying, for example.

Not only are CC foods lower in calories than fatty foods, but they are also more nutrient-dense – in other words they contain more vitamins and minerals, in particular iron and B vitamins. CC foods are also filling and they are ideal foods on which to snack – try wholemeal sandwiches, toast, fancy breads, fruit cakes (low-fat ones without icing), fruited buns and scones, teabreads and malt loaf. But Eat for Life Dieters cannot live on bread alone.

~ *Something more to chew over* ~

Rather than sprinkle bran on food, you can obtain fibre in a far more palatable form in starchy, CC foods. There is also more to fibre than the constipation-conquering role of insoluble fibre (bran) found in wheat, maize and rice. Soluble fibre in oats, beans, barley, rye, vegetables and some fruit has the added benefit of helping lower blood cholesterol. There are dozens of different types of fibre in CC foods, and they all work together to protect health.

~ *Take five* ~

In the following chapters you will discover how valuable fruit, vegetables and salads are. To meet Eat for Life Diet's CC goal, eat

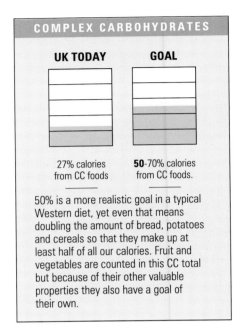

COMPLEX CARBOHYDRATES

UK TODAY — 27% calories from CC foods

GOAL — **50**-70% calories from CC foods.

50% is a more realistic goal in a typical Western diet, yet even that means doubling the amount of bread, potatoes and cereals so that they make up at least half of all our calories. Fruit and vegetables are counted in this CC total but because of their other valuable properties they also have a goal of their own.

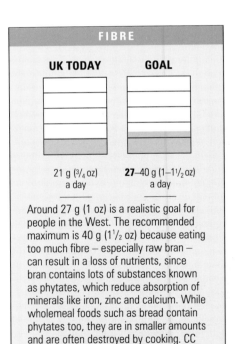

FIBRE

UK TODAY — 21 g (³/₄ oz) a day

GOAL — **27**–40 g (1–1¹/₂ oz) a day

Around 27 g (1 oz) is a realistic goal for people in the West. The recommended maximum is 40 g (1¹/₂ oz) because eating too much fibre – especially raw bran – can result in a loss of nutrients, since bran contains lots of substances known as phytates, which reduce absorption of minerals like iron, zinc and calcium. While wholemeal foods such as bread contain phytates too, they are in smaller amounts and are often destroyed by cooking. CC foods are also rich in vitamins, minerals and trace elements. Raw bran is not rich enough in minerals to compensate for its high phytate load.

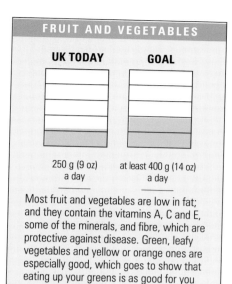

FRUIT AND VEGETABLES

UK TODAY	GOAL
250 g (9 oz) a day	at least 400 g (14 oz) a day

Most fruit and vegetables are low in fat; and they contain the vitamins A, C and E, some of the minerals, and fibre, which are protective against disease. Green, leafy vegetables and yellow or orange ones are especially good, which goes to show that eating up your greens is as good for you as everyone said.

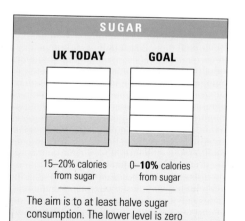

SUGAR

UK TODAY	GOAL
15–20% calories from sugar	0–**10%** calories from sugar

The aim is to at least halve sugar consumption. The lower level is zero which indicates that sugar is not needed in a healthy diet. Nevertheless, most people enjoy sweet things and don't want to give them up entirely, so at least make sure that sugar and sugary food account for no more than 10 per cent of your calorie intake.

400 g (14 oz, or nearly one pound) of fruit and vegetables a day. That's excluding potatoes, which are classed as starchy CC foods. This adds up to about five portions a day. Don't panic, it isn't as much as it sounds. Here's how to achieve it without becoming a fruit bat or eating a weird diet.

In a typical day you might have a glass of fruit juice for breakfast (count one), followed by an apple or a banana as a snack during the morning (count one for each piece of fruit). The Eat for Life Diet main meal of the day includes two portions of fresh, frozen or canned vegetables excluding potatoes (count one for each portion of veg, so that adds another two). And if you have an Eat for Life Diet fruit-based pudding you have added another portion, which brings you to your target of five – and you've simply eaten a normal diet.

If you don't eat meat, it is more important to include the 30 g (1 oz) a day of pulses, nuts and seeds as recommended by the WHO report. This provision was written in especially for vegetarians – more about that on pages 19–20.

~ Sugar – only on a Sunday ~

Sugar is for treats only in Eat for Life Diet, and, as with bread, it means adopting Continental eating habits. Even though there are many patisseries in France, and their equivalents in Italy and elsewhere, sweet cakes and pastries are not eaten on a daily basis like biscuits and confectionery are in Britain. In France these are seen as special treats. Most people choose a special cake from the patisserie for a treat at weekends, or when entertaining – which is exactly the Eat for Life Diet approach. Far from being a killjoy diet, it simply weans you off puddings with every meal, cookies with every coffee, and cakes or pastries with every cup of tea.

~ The fats of life ~

Oiling the works (with some polyunsaturated fats) is essential, but too much fat, especially saturated fat, increases the likelihood of heart disease and heart attacks. Cutting down on dietary fat reduces the risk of developing fat to avoid heart disease and some cancers and so is a number one health priority.

Reducing the amount of fat that is eaten is made easier by the

PORTIONS OF FRUIT AND VEGETABLES – AIM FOR FIVE A DAY

Each of those listed equals 1 portion, unless stated otherwise

FRUIT

Apple	
Avocado pear	$1/2$
Apricots, fresh or semi-dried	3–4
Banana	
Blackberries, raspberries, blackcurrants, cherries, gooseberries, stewed rhubarb or other cooked fruit	around 100 g (3$1/2$ oz)
Clementine or other citrus fruit such as mandarin, mineola, orange, tangerine, satsuma	
Damsons, greengages or other small plums	about 4
Dates, fresh or dried	4–6
Figs, fresh or dried	4
Grapefruit	$1/2$
Grapes	100 g (3$1/2$ oz)
Kiwifruit	2
Mango	$1/2$
Melon	175 g (6 oz)
Nectarine	
Passion fruit	4–5
Pawpaw	$1/2$
Peach	
Pear	
Pineapple	75–100 g (3–3$1/2$ oz)
Prunes	stewed: 6; semi-dried: 4
Sharon fruit	
Watermelon	200 g (7 oz)

FRUIT JUICE

1 citrus fruit squeezed
200 ml (7 fl oz) glass, which holds 200 g (7 oz) juice
Individual carton

VEGETABLES

Portions are around 75–100 g (3–3$1/2$ oz). Get to know how much this means in terms of 15 ml tablespoonfuls. You can eat more, of course; the list is just a rough guide to give you an idea of the variety of vegetables available.

Artichoke, globe	
Asparagus spears	5
Baked beans	
Broad beans	30 ml (2 tbsp)
French and runner beans	
Beansprouts	120 ml (8 tbsp)
Broccoli and calabrese	2 medium-large spears
Brussels sprouts	9–10
Cabbage	
Carrots, sliced	30 ml (2 tbsp)
Cauliflower	8 florets
Celery	3 sticks
Chickpeas	30–45 ml (2–3 tbsp)
Chinese leaf	2 large leaves
Coleslaw, low-fat	30 ml (2 tbsp)
Cucumber	5 cm (2 in) piece
Green banan	$1/2$
Leek	
Lentils	37–45 ml (2$1/2$–3 tbsp)
Lettuce	16 leaves
Marrow	
Mushrooms, poached	10
Mustard and cress	$1/2$ punnet equals $1/4$ portion
Okra	8 equal $1/4$ portion
Onion	1$1/2$–2
Parsnips	1 medium
Peas	45 ml (3 tbsp)
Pepper	
Plaintain	$1/3$–$1/2$
Ratatouille	45 ml (3 tbsp)
Sauerkraut	45 ml (3 tbsp)
Spinach	
Swede	
Sweetcorn	1 ear corn-on-the-cob
Tomatoes	1 large or 6 cherry
Turnip	
Watercress	1 bunch
Yam	

HIDDEN SUGAR		
	Sugar	
	ml	tsp
Chocolate milk shake (1 glass)	55–100	11–20
Chocolate fudge cake (slice)	55	11
Cola (1 glass)	45	9
Mars-type bar	45	9
Chocolate digestive biscuit	10	2
Tomato soup (half a can)	5	1
Allbran cereal (1 bowl)	5	1
Coco Pops (1 bowl)	15	3
Plain ice cream (1 portion)	10	2
Fruit yogurt (one small carton)	15	3

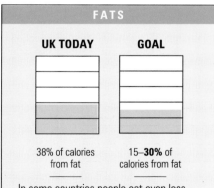

FATS	
UK TODAY	**GOAL**
38% of calories from fat	15–**30%** of calories from fat

In some countries people eat even less than 30 per cent of their calories as fat, but this amount would mean that the British diet would have to change drastically, so 30 per cent is a realistic target for the present. WHO thinks further benefits might be expected in the future by aiming for a fat intake approaching 15 per cent of total calories.

Eat for Life Diet's method of satisfying the appetite with CC foods and fruit and vegetables. By filling up on these you feel less need for fat.

The reason for replacing fatty foods is all to do with blood cholesterol. The higher the level of cholesterol in the blood, particularly if in addition to smoking and or high blood pressure, the greater the risk of developing heart disease.

Despite its bad reputation, cholesterol is essential for a healthy nervous system and for hormone production. The liver makes enough cholesterol for normal body functions, and it is carried in the bloodstream – hence blood cholesterol. Usually the body maintains a balance, producing more as it is needed and getting rid of excess, but sometimes the balance is upset.

If too many fatty foods are eaten, especially those containing saturated fats, there is a tendency for the cholesterol to build up in the artery walls, making them narrower and slowing down the supply of blood to the heart, or even cutting it off completely, at which point a heart attack occurs.

Diet alone is not the answer. As coronary heart disease has many causes, it is also important to try to do something about the other risk factors such as smoking, lack of exercise and raised blood pressure, if they apply to you. All of these things are within your control.

~ (M)eat to live? ~

There has been a lot of confusion about meat, especially red meat. You don't have to give up meat to have a healthy diet. There are lots of other fatty foods, including meat products, high-fat dairy foods and snacks, and are therefore the first priority when planning how to reduce your fat intake. Conversely, you don't have to eat meat to be healthy.

Red meat is a good source of iron and zinc and contains a useful amount of B vitamins, especially vitamin B12, which is found almost exclusively in animal products. Iron and zinc are more efficiently used by the body in the form found in meat. In animal products iron occurs in the 'haem' form; this is absorbed more easily by the body than the non-haem form of iron, which predominates in plant foods such as dark green vegetables, dried fruit, nuts and whole grains. Iron in vegetables is more easily absorbed when eaten with foods rich in vitamin C because vitamin C turns it into a form more readily usable by the body. On the other hand, drinking tea or, to a lesser extent, coffee with meals can reduce absorbtion of non-haem iron. These are not problems, just factors to be aware of if you don't eat meat or if you are cutting down on it. As regards zinc, vegetarians will find that wholemeal bread, pulses, eggs and nuts are all good sources.

Incidentally, if you do like meat, eat meat, not fat. Meat products such as burgers, pies, pâtés and sausages are notoriously high in saturated fat. Choose only lean cuts, and do not eat meat every day.

Liver may not be suitable for everyone. While it is a good source of iron, it is also very high in dietary cholesterol (as are kidneys and brains) and may need to be restricted in some diets. (See the advice about dietary cholesterol on pages 43–44 for more about this. Also, pregnant women have been warned not to eat it by the Department of Health because it might contain too much vitamin A, which can cause deformities in unborn babies. Animal feed suplemented with too much vitamin A has caused the problem. As this fat-soluble vitamin is stored in the liver it can build up to toxic levels. However once the feed problem is solved, this should no longer be an issue.

Among the healthiest diets in the world high-fat meats and cheeses are eaten only in small amounts. Often this is not for health reasons but simply because these foods are expensive or unavailable, especially in developing countries. The WHO report recommends that societies where a traditional diet still prevails should not give up their eating patterns and foods in favour of burgers, fried chicken and a Western way of eating.

In the West, we might do well to emulate the old tradition of 'fasting and feasting', killing the proverbial fatted calf only for a special occasion. Making meat more of a treat also means that quality can come before quantity, just as it does in the 28-day Slimming Plan. By better quality, we mean leaner meat from which you obtain more nutrients for less fat, and meat that has been produced with proper consideration of animal diet and welfare.

THE OLIVE OIL PHENOMENON

You may have heard that olive oil is better for you than sunflower oil. Scientists are reporting that monounsaturates (the main constituent fats of olive oil) can help lower blood cholesterol in the same way that polyunsaturates (found in sunflower, soya and corn oils) do. In southern Italy and Greece, where a lot of olive oil is used and little saturated fat is eaten, the rate of heart disease is very low, even though (as in Britain) around 40 per cent of calories in the diet come from fat, and many people are overweight.

Olive oil producers might say that this is all due to the monounsaturates in olive oil (see table on page 97). Indeed monounsaturates, like polyunsaturates, do help to lower levels of harmful blood cholesterol – but only as part of a low saturated-fat diet.

However, the low rate of heart disease where traditional Mediterranean diets are eaten could equally be due to the combination of all the healthy attributes of a diet rich in fruit and vegetables, high in CC food, in which fish replaces meat two or three times a week, and only small amounts of meat and dairy fats are eaten.

The most important way of reducing blood cholesterol levels, and thereby the risk of heart attack, is still to eat less fat, especially saturated fat – not to guzzle vast quantities of olive oil or sunflower oil. (For more details about how much polyunsaturated fat and dietary cholesterol you can eat, see page 44.)

~ Of fish and fowl ~

Lean meat also includes poultry and game. Poultry contains less fat than red meat; the fat is just under the skin and can easily be cut away when preparing or after cooking, before serving.

Eating more fish, at least twice a week, automatically reduces meat consumption, helping replace saturated fats with unsaturated fats. White fish is low in fat and high in vitamins and minerals. Oily fish has the added advantage of being rich in essential polyunsaturates called omega-3 fatty acids; these are different from the polyunsaturates found in vegetable oils. Omega-3 oils make the blood less sticky and therefore less likely to clot and cause a heart attack (see also notes in Appendix 1, page 148). It is unclear whether omega-3 oils can significantly reduce blood cholesterol, however, though they do seem to help lower triglycerides (another type of fat in the blood, the role of which in heart disease is not yet clear). Evidence of their ability to lower high blood pressure is poor. Obviously, for you to benefit, fish has to be a regular part of your diet.

~ Alive alive-O ~

Shellfish have had an undeservedly bad reputation recently with regard to cholesterol. Although they are high in dietary cholesterol, the British seaside favourites, cockles and mussels, winkles and whelks, are actually low in fat – as are prawns, shrimps and crab – and may therefore be eaten in moderation, because it is more important to reduce the amount of saturated fat than dietary cholesterol.

Dishes like *moules marinières* (mussels in white wine) are fine, whereas *moules à la creme* (mussels in cream sauce) obviously are not. Rich French seafood dishes tend to pile on the butter, tartare sauce, Béarnaise sauce and other mayonnaise-style sauces. Eat for Life Diet advocates instead plain grilled or barbecued fish, paellas, or seafood served in Thai, Chinese or Vietnamese dishes in which the 'sauce' is a broth-like soup containing lots of vegetables and sometimes noodles.

~ Dairy wise ~

While dairy products are a useful part of a healthy diet, contributing calcium and protein, moderation is the watchword. Medium- or low-fat versions of cheese, milk and yogurt are the Eat for Life Diet choice. Of course butter and cream do not have to be given up entirely, just limited to treats, where they would be missed the most.

Choose low-fat versions of milk and yogurt, or on special occasions Greek yogurt instead of cream. And while eggs are nutritious and convenient, the yolks are high in dietary cholesterol. The general consensus is that you should have no more than about four a week, including those used in cooking, because they are high in dietary cholesterol.

CHOICE CHEESES

Low-fat cheese (in which 25–45% or fewer of the calories are from fat): fromage frais, quark and similar low-fat soft white cheeses

Medium-fat cheese (in which 25-45% of the calories are from fat): cottage cheese (35%)

High-fat cheese (in which 60% or more of the calories are from fat): Cheddar and other hard cheeses, blue cheeses, cream cheeses, Edam, Brie, Camembert, goat's cheese

~ Salt – who needs it? ~

You will get all the salt you need from bread, cereals, fruit and vegetables: you don't have to lift a finger for the salt cellar. Today most people eat twice as much salt as they need, most coming from processed foods. The reason for halving it is that eating too much salt is linked with high blood pressure (though whether it actually causes it is still controversial). High blood pressure in turn increases the risk of stroke and heart attack. Adding more salt to food may also exacerbate existing health problems. (For more information about salt and high blood pressure, see pages 46–47.)

~ Protein needs ~

Cereals and pulses are the main foods eaten by the majority of the world's population. In the affluent West it's often forgotten that even cereals and vegetables provide protein. We think of protein only in terms of meat, fish, eggs and dairy produce, yet as part of a varied diet vegetables and cereals can provide 10–15 per cent of calories in the form of protein.

Sportsmen and women no longer believe that it's necessary to eat meat to be fit and strong. As long as enough calories are consumed in a typical Western diet, protein needs will look after themselves. In fact, eating more than 15 per cent of calories as protein may be harmful, as it promotes calcium loss from bones, which may lead to osteoporosis, and it also puts the kidneys under strain.

MEAT AND FISH

Low-fat meat and fish (in which 25% or less of the calories are from fat) MAY BE EATEN OFTEN

Poached or steamed white fish

Roast chicken or turkey, without skin

Lean roast beef

Canned fish in brine

Prawns

Scallops

Medium-fat meat and fish (in which 45% or less of the calories are from fat) MAY BE EATEN QUITE OFTEN

Grilled or steamed trout

Salmon

Lean boiled ham

Lean roast duck, without skin

Lean roast leg of pork

Lean roast venison

Stewed offal

Sardines and pilchards in tomato sauce

Lean grilled pork chop, without fat

Stewed rabbit

Stewed lean beef

Medium–high. fat meat (in which around 60% of the calories are from fat) MAY BE EATEN RARELY AND IN SMALL QUANTITIES

Bacon

Mince

Chops

Gammon – meat and fat

Liver sausage

Sausages

Salami

Luncheon meat

Pork pie and other meat pies

Pâté

Scotch eggs

In the 1960s and '70s vegetarians followed complicated charts showing how to combine in one meal foods from two or three of the four basic groups of vegetarian protein foods. Now we know that all this is unnecessary. However, it is a good idea for vegetarians (and meat-eaters as well) to eat different sources of protein each day as it is unwise to be over-reliant on one food. Also vegetarians can easily eat too much saturated fat if they rely heavily on cheese and eggs.

For those with an academic interest, the vegetarian groups of protein are: (1) beans and pulses, (2) nuts and seeds, (3) cereals and grains and (4) milk, cheese and yogurt.

Parents who worry when children decide to go vegetarian, whether it is for days, weeks or years, can be reassured that their health is not in danger if the Eat for Life Diet's basic guidelines are followed. (See pages 51–58 for details about the Junior Eating Plan.) Vegetarian options are also given in the eating plans and the 28-day Slimming Plan.

~ The best of all worlds ~

There's a lot to be learnt from watching Chinese people shop – whether in Szechuan, Soho or San Francisco. Traditionally, CC foods (rice or noodles) are chosen first, making up the bulk of the diet. Next the greens are chosen – Chinese markets and supermarkets have a wonderful array of vegetables. Last to go in the shopping basket is the meat or fish: perhaps a few prawns, some spare ribs or a small amount of pork or poultry.

By adopting this system of shopping and eating, CC foods easily become a major part of the diet. First choose your CC foods (for information see recipe section begining on page 97) and plan the rest of the menu from there.

The system works well with dishes from most cuisines and cultures – even the ultimate convenience food, the sandwich. From now on, make it a doorstep sandwich every time. Buy unsliced bread and cut it thick, then add lots of salad and finally a small amount of lean meat, fish or low-fat cheese. You don't even need to butter the bread – the salad will add enough moisture – but if you do, use just a small amount of unsaturated fat.

The type of sandwich found on Wall Street, which contains a huge amount of pastrami spilling out of thin slices of rye bread, with a side order of coleslaw swimming in high-calorie mayonnaise, is an Eat for Life Dieter's nightmare. Much better to follow the lead of the west coast, and choose a California-style sandwich. In this the toasted bread is cut as thick as a baguette, unbuttered and filled with lots of green salad and a moderate portion of char-grilled meat or fish, with more green salad on the side.

There are lots more examples of CC eating from around the world. When in Rome, for example, go for the pasta first and then the sauce. Choose tomato sauces (not fatty and floury sauces like the British macaroni-cheese), or choose pasta that is stuffed with spinach and medium-fat ricotta. A small amount of Parmesan cheese is sprinkled on top. To an Italian – and an Eat for Life Dieter – the pasta is more important than the sauce.

~ Cooking the healthiest diet in the world ~

Quick preparation, just ahead of use, helps prevent loss of vitamins and minerals. When boiling vegetables, use as little water as possible, adding the vegetables only after the water has come to the boil. Do not overcook them. Avoid cooking methods that use lots of fat, especially saturated fat (palm oil, coconut oil, lard, suet, butter, hard margarine, dripping). Instead, opt for grilling, steaming, boiling, stir-frying, poaching, baking, casseroling, barbecuing, microwaving. For more tips, ideas and recipes see the Eat for Life Diet's Eating Plans (pages 65–84) and recipes (pages 97–146).

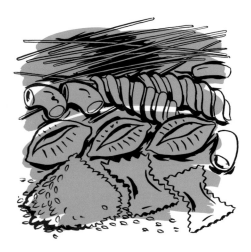

Superfoods and Supernutrients

t's a popular view that no single food is either healthy or unhealthy. It's the sum total of the diet that is either healthy or unhealthy. However in the context of the Eat for Life Diet, some foods contribute more to healthy eating and living than others.

Although certain foods have been identified as being better than others, they still have to be eaten as part of a balanced diet, which means eating a variety of foods. No matter how super a food, no one food contains all nutrients. Different foods are rich in different nutrients.

That said, many fruits, vegetables, and CC foods contain special combinations of vitamins and minerals that are associated with a lower risk of heart disease and some diet-related cancers. We have called these foods 'superfoods' and they are central to Eat for Life Diet.

~ Do you eat enough superfoods? ~

Fruit, vegetables, salad, bread, wholegrain cereals, potatoes, pulses, fish, low-fat dairy produce and lean meats are Eat for Life Diet's superfoods. If you are now thinking, 'I eat them, so I'm all right, I don't have to read any further', hold on – not so fast! Yes, you may be eating these foods, but do you eat the right amounts of them?

Superfoods are superior to many others because they are nutrient dense. This means that every mouthful contains the maximum amount of nutrients (vitamins, minerals) and fibre for the number of calories. However, in the Eat for Life Diet we concentrate on foods – and superfoods in particular – rather than on nutrients, because it is food that we eat, enjoy and shop for, rather than the vitamins and minerals it contains.

The value of superfoods is apparent when they are compared to foods such as sugar, alcohol, some types of fat, and confectionery, all of which contain a lot of calories but very few nutrients.

Although we all know that we need vitamins and minerals, we perhaps forget sometimes that they are essential for health. They are needed for protection against disease (see below) and for the millions of chemical reactions in the body that control everything from digestion of food and absorption of its energy to the building of new cells, the working of muscles, and whether or not we have clear, healthy skin and a healthy smile.

Eating cakes, confectionery, meat pies, chips, sausages or sweets might provide you with enough calories but you could end up suffering from malnutrition while, paradoxically, being overweight. This is a difficult concept to grasp when we are used to equating malnutrition with the starving people in Third World countries. But it is possible to be overweight and under-nourished.

~ Protecting against diseases ~

Superfoods have been associated with a reduced risk of diet-related diseases, such as the following. (For more information, see pages 43–50.)

- Eating fruit and vegetables frequently, in particular broccoli, cabbage and other dark green leafy veg, may lower the risk of diet-related cancers.
- The many different types of fibre in CC foods are associated with lower rates of diet-related cancers, diverticulosis and constipation.
- CC foods probably also help reduce the risk of heart disease and some diabetes.
- Water-soluble fibres in oatbran, beans and some fruit are associated with reducing blood cholesterol levels.

~ What superfoods have to offer ~

The specific components that give superfoods their protective powers have not yet been established beyond doubt, but the current evidence overwhelmingly suggests we would do well to eat more of them.

Apricots, peaches and nectarines are rich in beta carotene and vitamin C. Dried apricots lose their vitamin C but are rich in iron and fibre. Plant food sources of iron are most easily absorbed when eaten with vitamin C foods like citrus fruit juice, green leafy vegetables or berries.

Breast milk is the ideal superfood for babies. For best quality breast milk, mum's diet needs to be rich in superfoods and supernutrients. She also needs to eat a little extra overall and take plenty of rest and relaxation.

Broccoli, brussels sprouts and cabbage are rich sources of carotene and vitamin C, and some vitamin E. Vitamin C is destroyed by over-cooking, and all vitamins are reduced by leaving cut vegetables exposed to air if prepared too long in advance of eating or cooking. The outer, darker leaves are the most nutrient dense and contain the most fibre. Other green leafy vegetables such as spinach and watercress, are also rich in vitamin C and carotene and contain some vitamin E and folic acid (a B vitamin). Brussels sprouts, cabbage and spinach also contain vitamin B6.

Carrots are an excellent source of carotene, particulaly when raw. Old carrots contain more carotene when cooked than young.

Citrus fruit such as oranges, lemons, limes and grapefruit are good sources of vitamin C. Some contain a little carotene with traces of folic acid.

Oats and beans contain gummy soluble types of fibre that may lower the levels of harmful cholesterol in the bloodstream. It is also thought that they may regulate blood sugar levels, smoothing out the 'ups and downs' by providing 'slow-release' energy, although there is not enough evidence to be conclusive about this.

Oily fish such as herring, mackerel, sardines, salmon, trout and sprats provide fat-soluble vitamins. Fish oil is a source of polyunsaturates called omega-3 fatty acids. These contribute to changes in blood, by making it less 'sticky' and so less likely to clot, thereby reducing the risk of heart attack and stroke. They are vital also for the development of the brain, proving the old adage that fish is good for the brain.

Olive oil (see also page 20) contains mainly monounsaturates, which can help lower blood cholesterol levels, like polyunsaturates – and some types of olive oil taste better than polyunsaturated oils. Avocados, most nuts (especially almonds and peanuts, but not walnuts or coconuts), peanut oil and canola oil (which is manufactured from a type of rapeseed oil) are other good sources of monounsaturates.

Lentils are a good source of B vitamins and, like oats and beans (and some fruit and vegetables), they may also regulate blood sugar levels. A good source of vegetarian protein.

Nuts are a good source of vitamin E and many B vitamins. Rich in oil, they are also high in calories – a watchpoint for slimmers. Brazil nuts, cashews, hazelnuts, walnuts and peanuts are all good sources of polyunsaturates. Coconuts are virtually devoid of vitamins, and coconut oil (as well as palm oil) is unusual among vegetable oils in being high in saturated fat.

~ Protective foods ~

The idea of protective foods is not new. Some readers may have come across World War II leaflets from the Ministry of Food which spoke about 'foods for protection against ill health', suggesting people eat more of these foods. In particular, the advice which still holds good today in the light of new scientific evidence is that some foods from each group – vitamin A, B vitamins and vitamin C – should be eaten on a daily basis.

Few rosehips are eaten these days, but we agree with daily portions of foods from each of these groups, with the riders that the milk and cheese be low-fat and that polyunsaturated fats be used for spreading and cooking in order to cut down on saturated fat. During the war, flour and bread (the National Loaf) were 81 per cent extraction: brown, but not quite wholemeal. In fact, the diet was one of the healthiest Britain has known – but it was not well-liked because of its associations with deprivation. Now that food is in good supply, however, there is a far greater choice than ever before in each of the above categories (see pages 31–38).

~ ACE eating ~

Scientists have not established conclusively what it is in fruit and vegetables that is so beneficial, but one theory suggests that it is actually the combination of nutrients working together.

A lot of interest centres on beta carotene (see box), and vitamins C and E. These vitamins, which often occur in clusters in fruit and vegetables, are found in berries, orange and yellow fruit, and green vegetables. What we have called 'ACE eating' is about eating enough vitamin A, C and E. There are still many people who could eat more of the foods that contain these nutrients. Both vitamins A and C are needed for a healthy immune system, which protects the body against infection.

WORLD WAR II PROTECTIVE FOODS

Vitamin A	B vitamins	Vitamin C
milk	peas	green vegetables
cheese	beans	
green vegetables	lentils	root vegetables
	nuts	
butter	bread	potatoes
margarine	flour	oranges
eggs	oatmeal	blackcurrants
carrots		tomatoes
liver		rosehips

BETA CAROTENE

Beta carotene is the pigment that gives green, yellow and orange fruit and vegetables their colour. In the body it is turned into vitamin A, so it is known as a vitamin A precursor. Along with other nutrients it is being studied for its protective powers.

In addition, all three vitamins protect us through their antioxidant powers. Antioxidants help prevent the oxidation of fats, which turns food rancid and can have similar destructive effects in the body. While we don't literally turn rancid, or even rusty like the oxidation reaction between oxygen and some metals, oxidation can be seriously harmful to humans. That's why there is such a lot of interest in antioxidant nutrients.

~ Inactivating free radicals ~

The importance of the vitamins' antioxidant power lies in their ability to neutralise 'free radicals', which are highly active and damaging and have consequently been the focus of much scientific attention over the last ten years.

Free radicals may initiate some cancers and heart disease. They are a by-product of normal cell activity, but they can also be created by pollutants such as chemicals, cigarette smoke and radiation (i.e. X rays). They are very reactive molecules because they are one electron short (electrons are usually paired), so they grab an electron from another molecule. This disturbs the chemical balance by making another electron a single unit and setting up a chain reaction, rather like a line of falling dominoes.

Although free radicals exist only momentarily, they need to be dealt with because, inside cells, they are capable of damaging DNA, the genetic material in cells, which can produce potentially carcinogenic (cancer-causing) cells. And they may set up chain reactions in atherosclerosis (arterial plaque) that lead to further narrowing of the arteries, increasing the risk of heart attacks.

To counter the effects of free radicals, we need antioxidants, such as vitamin A in the form of beta carotene, vitamin C and vitamin E. They inactivate the free radicals by donating electrons, thereby preventing the destructive chain reactions that could otherwise lead to cancer or atherosclerosis. Once they have donated their electrons, antioxidant vitamins then decay harmlessly.

Cells are also equipped with defences such as antioxidant enzymes made from selenium and other trace minerals. Although much of this remains to be confirmed, it may explain the difference between the large amount of heart disease in the UK in comparison with other European countries where fat intake is fairly high but where, unlike in Britain, a lot of fruit and vegetables are eaten.

SELENIUM – ANOTHER ACE NUTRIENT?

Antioxidant enzymes are formed from minerals such as selenium, iron and zinc, and trace elements such as manganese and copper. Selenium in particular has been singled out as an effective antioxidant. Areas of the UK (East Anglia and Scotland) and elsewhere in the world where the soil is rich in selenium have been linked with longevity. These observations have not been fully tested, however, and scientists are still studying the role of selenium – which is toxic in large doses – in protecting against disease.

~ Cracking the code ~

Everyone needs vitamins and minerals to protect against disease and be fit and healthy. Some people need more than others, however. Individual prescriptions can only be worked out after a battery of scientific tests. But nutritional scientists have looked at the general needs of different groups of people in different conditions and come up with categories for various age groups. Until recently there were RDA (Recommended Daily Amounts) of nutrients for people in the UK. You have probably noticed on nutritional labelling of food that particular foods give you a certain percentage of your daily requirement of various vitamins and minerals.

RDAs have now been superseded by new standards called Dietary Reference Values, or DRVs. These were described in the British government report *Dietary Reference Values for Food Energy and Nutrients for the UK*, a report produced by a committee of experts who made up a COMA (Committee on Medical Aspects of Food Policy) panel on the subject. Full details are in Appendix 2 but it's useful to know some of the new terminology about vitamins and minerals as it might appear on food packaging.

Dietary Reference Values (DRVs) is a blanket term for any of the following. Any one DRV (i.e. nutrient) depends on all the others being met; no single DRV can be taken in isolation.

Estimated Average Requirement (EAR) is an assessment of the average requirement or need for food energy, or for a particular nutrient. Many people will need more than the average and many will need less.

Reference Nutrient Intake (RNI) is the amount of a nutrient which is sufficient for almost every individual. It is the equivalent of the old RDA. This level of intake is much higher than a lot of people need.

Lower Reference Nutrient Intake (LRNI) is the amount of a nutrient considered to be sufficient for the small number of people with low needs. Most people will need more than the LRNI if they are to eat enough. If people consistently eat fewer vitamins and minerals than the LRNI they are at high risk of deficiency of that nutrient.

A PLEA TO COOKS

In the middle of all this scientific information, let's not forget that the Eat for Life Diet is about food. Vegetables in particular have for too long been mere garnishes to meat or fish. Now it is time to make them the pièce de résistance and treat them as the main ingredient in all meals and snacks.

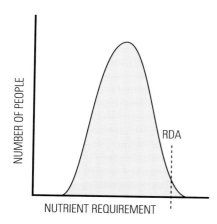

The first graph shows the range of needs for a nutrient (vitamin or mineral). Some people need very little, most people fall somewhere in the middle (the hump of the distribution curve) and some people need a lot. The old RDA was set at the top end to cover most people's needs.

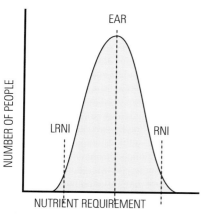

The second graph shows the three new values in their positions in the distribution curve.

Safe Intake is the amount given when there is insufficient information to estimate requirements. The safe intake is judged to be adequate for almost everyone's needs, and not large enough to cause illness or undesirable side effects.

To understand the DRVs it's helpful to look at the graphs on this page.

~ ACE foods ~

The $64,000 question for most people will be, 'How much of each vitamin or mineral do I need?' While Eat for Life Diet can't give individual prescriptions, the following is a useful guide based on the British government's Dietary Reference Values. It gives a brief outline to needs for each nutrient and the best food sources – eat more of these foods. For the full DRV table see Appendix 2.

The 'top ten' sources below are a guide to which foods are good sources of nutrients. They are not there for readers to measure out exact quantities in order to achieve exact intakes. **Nutrient content was calculated in metric (g). Imperial figures are approximations to the original metric.**

Vitamin C – How Much?

Vitamin C is widely available in fruit and vegetables. Humans cannot make vitamin C in the body, so it has to be eaten. It is known that 10 mg a day is enough to prevent scurvy, but not enough for vitamin C to be measurable in the body. Intakes of about 30 mg a day are needed for it to be measurable and up to 70mg for it to reach maximum concentration. As significant amounts are present at 40 mg per day intake the EAR has been set at that level. The DRV report says there is no evidence that 1 gram or more a day of vitamin C offers protection against the common cold, cancer or other disorders. Taking too much vitamin C may cause diarrhoea and kidney stones.

For Dietary Reference Values for vitamin C see Appendix 2

Top ten sources of vitamin C per portion

Vitamin C is expressed as milligrams (mg) to the nearest 0.5. The food is fresh and raw unless stated otherwise. Where cooked, no sugar is added. Juices are unsweetened. The amounts given are standard portions.

Guava 217 mg per 90 g (3^1/$_4$ oz), blackcurrants 210 mg per 140g (5 oz), Pawpaw (papaya) 102 mg per 140 g (5 oz) (half a fruit), orange juice (canned) 70 mg per 200 g (7 oz), strawberries 67 mg per 113 g (4 oz), orange 64 per 170 g (6 oz), grapefruit juice (canned) 56 mg per 200 g (7 oz), mango (half a fruit) 48 mg per 160 g (5^3/$_4$ oz), spinach 46 mg per 90 g (3^1/$_4$ oz), melon (honeydew) 45 mg per 180 g (6^1/$_2$ oz).

Vitamin E – How Much?

Despite all the publicity about fruit and vegetables containing lots of vitamin E, this does not seem to be the case. Vegetable oils and starchy CC foods are better sources of vitamin E.

The amount you need of this antioxidant vitamin depends on how much polyunsaturated fat you eat because vitamin E is needed to prevent polyunsaturates being oxidised. As polyunsaturate intake varies a lot, no DRV has been set for vitamin E, but the 'safe' intake is 4 mg a day for men and 3 mg for women. However, this is not to say you can't eat more. According to the DRV panel, few adverse effects have been reported on doses up to 3,200 mg per day.

Top ten sources of vitamin E per portion

Vitamin E is expressed as milligrams (mg) to the nearest 0.5. The food is fresh and raw unless stated otherwise. Where cooked, no sugar is added. Juices are unsweetened. The amounts given are standard portions.

Blackberries (stewed) 4 mg per 140 g (5 oz), vegetable oils, about 6 mg per 15 ml (1 tbsp), asparagus 3 mg per 125 g (4^1/$_2$ oz), tuna in oil 3 mg per 45 g (1^1/$_2$ oz), kedgeree 3 mg per 300 g (11 oz), avocado 2 mg per 75 g (2^3/$_4$ oz) (half an avocado), muesli 2 mg per 70 g (2^1/$_2$ oz), naan bread 2 mg per 160 g (5^3/$_4$ oz) (one large bread), risotto (plain) 2 mg per 250 g (9 oz), nuts (peanuts, hazelnuts, almonds) about 2 mg per 25 g (scant 1 oz) portion. NB Margarine varies between brands but provides around 0.8 mg per 10 g (^{1}/$_3$ oz) average portion used to spread a piece of bread.

Beta Carotene – How Much?

Beta carotene is widely available in fruit and vegetables, particularly green and yellow ones. It is turned into vitamin A (retinol) in the body. There are no recommendations in the DRVs about the proportion of vitamin A which should be derived from beta carotene and the proportion from retinol (vitamin A foods).

ARE YOU FRUITY ENOUGH?

Sixty-two per cent of people claim to eat fresh fruit once a day or more, 30 per cent only once a week, 3 per cent only once a month, 2 per cent less than once a month, 2 per cent never and, extraordinarily enough, 1 per cent don't know.

Fifty-eight per cent of people eat fresh vegetables once a day or more, 36 per cent only once a week, 1 per cent only once month, 1 per cent less than once a month and 3 per cent of people never eat fresh vegetables. Once again, that 1 per cent don't know.

Eat Life for Life Dieters eat fruit and vegetables every day.

Although scientists have some evidence that beta carotene is protective against cancer, they do not yet know enough to make specific recommendations on how much we need. High intakes of beta carotene from food, on the other hand, do not seem to be harmful. They can turn the skin an orangey colour but, as far as it is known, that is all.

Top ten sources of beta carotene per portion

Beta carotene is expressed as micrograms (μg). The food is fresh and raw unless stated otherwise. Where cooked, no sugar is added. Juices are unsweetened. The amounts given are standard portions.

Mixed vegetable curry 10,350 μg per 300 g (11 oz), carrots (old, boiled) 10,200 μg per 85 g (3 oz), carrots (old) 7,200 μg per 60 g ($2^1/_4$ oz), spinach (boiled) 5,400 μg per 90 g ($3^1/_4$ oz), sweet potaotes (boiled) 4,800 μg per 120 g ($4^1/_4$ oz), spinach 4,374 μg per 90 g ($3^1/_4$ oz), spring greens (boiled) 3,600 μg per 90 g ($3^1/_4$ oz), cantaloupe melon 3,000 μg per 150 g ($5^1/_4$ oz), ox liver (stewed) 2,186 μg per 142 g (5 oz), mango 1,920 μg per 160 g ($5^3/_4$ oz) (half a fruit).

Vitamin A – How Much?

Vitamin A is measured as retinol-equivalent, while beta carotene has to be turned into retinol in the body. Eating too much vitamin A over a period of time may be dangerous, as it can lead to liver and bone damage, especially in children and pregnant women. Regular intakes should not exceed 7,500 μg for women and 9,000 μg for men. A far lower limit of 3,500 μg is recommended for pregnant women because it may cause birth defects. (More about this is on page 20.)

For Dietary Reference Values for vitamin A see Appendix 2

Top ten sources of vitamin A per portion

Vitamin A is expressed as micrograms (μg) of retinol (vitamin A equivalent). The food is fresh and raw unless stated otherwise. Where cooked, no sugar is added. Juices are unsweetened. The amounts given are standard portions.

Liver (ox, stewed) 28,906 μg per 142 g (5 oz), chicken curry (without bones) 7,770 μg per 300 g (11 oz), mixed vegetable curry 2,139 μg per 300 g (11 oz), carrots (old, boiled) 1,700 μg per 85 g (3 oz), spinach (boiled) 900 μg per 90 g ($3^1/_4$ oz), herring curry

803 µg per 300 g (11 oz), sweet potatoes (boiled) 800 µg per 120 g (4¹/₄ oz), haddock curry 722 µg per 300 g (11 oz), spring greens (boiled) 600 µg per 90 g (3¹/₄ oz), Spanish omelette 501 µg per 150 g (5¹/₄ oz).

~ *The B Group* ~

ACE eating to ensure an adequate beta carotene (vitamin A), vitamin C and vitamin E intake is important, and is probably the key to much disease prevention, but other nutrients are also essential. The B vitamins found in CC foods, meat and milk, for example, are vital for the nervous system, and release of energy from food during digestion.

Thiamin (vitamin B1) – How Much?

Thiamin is needed for the release of energy from food. Because it is needed for burning calories, the amount required depends on the amount of food eaten (see Appendix 2). No extra thiamin is needed during pregnancy or breastfeeding. Intake is limited to three grams a day because in the long-term, more could be harmful.

For Dietary Reference Values for thiamin see Appendix 2

Top ten sources of thiamin (vitamin B1) per portion

Thiamin is expressed as milligrams (mg). The food is fresh and raw unless stated otherwise. Where cooked, no sugar is added. Juices are unsweetened. The amounts given are standard portions.
Oxtail soup 1.5 mg per 220 g (7³/₄ oz), gammon rashers (grilled, lean only) 1.5 mg per 170 g (6 oz), cod roe (fried) 1.5 mg per 116 g (4 oz), gammon joint (boiled, lean only) 1 mg per 170 g (6 oz), pork chops (loin, grilled, lean only) 1 mg per 100 g (3¹/₂ oz), breakfast cereals such as Start 0.6 mg per 40 g (1¹/₂ oz), Farmhouse Bran 0.5 mg per 40 g (1¹/₂ oz), bulghur wheat 0.5 mg per 100 g (3¹/₂ oz), Vital (calcium fortified milk) 0.5 mg per 146g (5¹/₄ oz), wholemeal pasta (boiled) 0.5 mg per 35 g (1¹/₄ oz), brown rice 0.4 mg per 60 g (2 oz).

Riboflavin (vitamin B2) – How Much?

Like thiamin, riboflavin is needed for energy release. For sedentary people the amount depends on the number of calories eaten, while active people need more. Riboflavin overdose is unlikely because it is not easily absorbed by the body.

For Dietary Reference Values for riboflavin see Appendix 2

Top ten sources of riboflavin per portion

Riboflavin is expressed as milligrams (mg). The food is fresh and raw unless stated otherwise. Where cooked, no sugar is added. Juices are unsweetened. The amounts given are standard portions. Ox liver (stewed) 5 mg per 142 g (5 oz), cod roe (dried) 1 mg per 116 g (4 oz), ox heart (stewed) 1 mg per 85 g (3 oz), mackerel (fried) 1 mg per 200 g (7 oz), Calcia (fortified milk) 1 mg per 146 g (5¼ oz), breakfast cereals such as Shreddies 1 mg per 35 g (1¼ oz), scrambled eggs (without milk) 0.4 mg per 100 g (3½ oz), gammon rashers (grilled, lean only) 0.5 mg per 170 g (6 oz), whole milk fruit yogurt 0.5 mg per 150 g (5¼ oz), herring roe (fried) 0.5 mg per 85 g (3 oz), low-fat natural yogurt 0.4 mg per 150 g (5½ oz).

Niacin (vitamin B3) – How Much?

This is another B vitamin involved in release of energy where the amount needed depends on the calories eaten. The body can also make niacin from some protein foods. Very high doses, of 3–6g per day, can cause liver damage. Doses of 200 mg a day can cause flushing, which is harmless but is not found with lower intakes. Breastfeeding women may need extra niacin.

For Dietary Reference Values for niacin see Appendix 2

Top ten sources of niacin per portion

Niacin is expressed as milligrams (mg) of nicotinic acid (niacin equivalent). The food is fresh and raw unless stated otherwise. Where cooked, no sugar is added. Juices are unsweetened. The amounts given are standard portions.
Mackerel (fried) 17.5 mg per 200 g (7 oz), pig liver (stewed) 16 mg per 142 g (5 oz), ox liver (stewed) 14 mg per 142 g (5 oz), herring curry 13 mg per 300 g (11 oz), haddock curry 13 mg per 300 g (11 oz), gammon rashers (grilled, lean only) 12 mg per 170 g

(6 oz), chicken curry (without bones) 12 mg per 300 g (11 oz), turkey (roast, light meat) 9 mg per 90 g (3¼ oz), chicken (roast, dark meat) 8.5 mg per 140 g (5 oz), sardines (canned in oil) 8 mg per 100 g (3½ oz).

Vitamin B6 – How Much?

The amount needed is related to protein intake. The DRVs have been worked out on the current protein intake in the UK. Extra B6 is not needed for pregnancy or breastfeeding. According to the DRV report, oral contraceptives do not increase the need for B6, contrary to popular belief. However, very high levels of vitamin B6 can counter some effects of the pill in some women. High intakes, between 50 mg and 7 g per day, can impair nerve function.

For Dietary Reference Values for vitamin B6 see Appendix 2

Top ten sources of vitamin B6 per portion

Vitamin B6 is expressed as milligrams (mg). The food is fresh and raw unless stated otherwise. Where cooked, no sugar is added. Juices are unsweetened. The amounts given are standard portions. Plantain (green, fried) 2 mg per 200 g (7 oz), mackerel (fried) 1.5mg per 200 g (7 oz), liver (pig, stewed) 1 mg per 142 g (5 oz), breakfast cereal such as Start 1 mg per 40 g (1½ oz), salmon (steamed, flesh only) 0.5 mg per 100 g (3½ oz), liver (ox, stewed) 0.5 mg per 142 g (5 oz), saithe (steamed with bones) 0.5 mg per 120 g (4¼ oz), gammon rashers (grilled, lean only) 0.5 mg per 170 g (6 oz), cod (grilled) 0.5 mg per 150 g (5¼ oz), bananas 0.5 mg per 100 g (3½ oz).

Vitamin B12 – How Much?

Vitamin B12 is needed to help protect the nerves and to protect against anaemia. B12 works in particular with folic acid. High intakes are not dangerous. Vegetarians and vegans need to pay attention to their intake as B12 is found almost exclusively in animal products.

For Dietary Reference Values for vitamin B12 see Appendix 2

Top ten sources of vitamin B12 per portion

Vitamin B12 is expressed as micrograms (μg). The food is fresh and raw unless stated otherwise. Where cooked, no sugar is added.

Juices are unsweetened. The amounts given are standard portions. Liver (ox, stewed) 156 µg per 142 g (5 oz), lamb kidney (fried) 71 µg per 90 g ($3^1/_4$ oz), sardines (canned in oil) 28 µg per 100 g ($3^1/_2$ oz), mackerel (fried) 24 µg per 200 g (7 oz), cod roe (fried) 12 µg per 116 g (4 oz), ox heart (stewed) 12 µg per 116 g (4 oz), rabbit (stewed with bones) 10 µg per 85 g (3 oz), herring (grilled with bones) 9 µg per 119 g ($4^1/_4$ oz), turkey (roast, dark meat) 3 µg per 90 g ($3^1/_4$ oz), cod (grilled) 3 µg per 150 g ($5^1/_4$ oz), Yeast extract 0.05 µg per 10 g ($^1/_3$ oz).

Folates – How Much?

Folates is the name given to a group of substances made from folic acid, another B vitamin. DRVs are based on the amounts of folate in food needed to maintain 'normal' stores in the liver and red blood cells. Pregnant women need extra folate in late pregnancy. Evidence shows that folic acid supplements taken before pregnancy can prevent spina bifida in babies among women who have already had a pregnancy affected by neural tube defects. For affected women one 5 mg tablet a day before starting a further pregnancy is recommended. All women who are likely to become pregnant would benefit from increased intake of folic acid, and a government committee was being set up at the end of 1991 to look into how best to increase women's intake of this nutrient. In the meantime it would be prudent for women to eat foods rich in folic acid. Although liver is a good source, women who may become pregnant are at present advised not to eat it (see page 20).

For Dietary Reference Values for folates see Appendix 2

Top ten sources of folic acid per portion

Folic acid is expressed as micrograms (µg). The food is fresh and raw unless stated otherwise. Where cooked, no sugar is added. Juices are unsweetened. The amounts given are standard portions. Liver (ox, stewed) 411 µg per 142 g (5 oz), spinach (boiled) 126 µg per 90 g ($3^1/_4$ oz), spinach 110 µg per 90 g ($3^1/_4$ oz), breakfast cereals such as corn flakes 100 µg per 40 g ($1^1/_2$ oz), endive (lettuce) 99 µg per 30 g (1 oz), spring greens (boiled) 99 µg per 90 g ($3^1/_4$ oz), Brussels sprouts (boiled) 78 µg per 90 g ($3^1/_4$ oz), cheese and tomato pizza 64 µg per 280 g (10 oz), chicken curry (with bones) 60 µg per 300 g (11 oz), cabbage (red/white) 54 µg per 60 g ($2^1/_4$ oz), melon (honeydew) 54 µg per 180 g ($6^1/_2$ oz).

SPUD YOU LIKE?

We are buying fewer potatoes, greens and root vegetables for consumption at home in the UK. The decline in family meat-and-two-veg meals is blamed for the decrease in the last 20 years from 63.5 kg (140 lb) of potatoes per person per year to 54 kg (120 lb); from 17 kg (38 lb) of root veg to 12 kg (26 lb); and from 14 kg (30 lb) of green veg to 13 kg (28 lb). The Eat for Life Diet wants you to change all that and eat more potatoes and starchy root vegetables.

~ Don't underestimate D ~

Although we talk about 'vitamin D', it is in fact a hormone needed for the absorption of calcium, which is essential for bones and teeth. It is nicknamed the 'sunshine vitamin' because most vitamin D is made in the skin by the action of sun – not sunbathing, just natural daylight.

Vitamin D – How Much?

Vitamin D is found only in a few foods, yet it is still important for strong teeth and bones because it is needed for calcium and phosphorus absorption. Toddlers and children who don't eat enough may develop rickets – those mainly at risk are in the Asian community because the traditional diet is low in calcium and there is limited exposure to daylight. In adults deficiency can lead to osteomalacia; similar to rickets, it is a softening of the bones owing to a lack of vitamin D. Children are more at risk from high intakes, of 50 µg per day, than adults.

For Dietary Reference Values for vitamin D see Appendix 2

Top ten sources of vitamin D per portion

Vitamin D is expressed as micrograms (µg). The food is fresh and raw unless stated otherwise. Where cooked, no sugar is added. Juices are unsweetened. The amounts given are standard portions. Mackerel (fried) 42 µg per 200 g (7 oz), herring (grilled) 21 µg per 85 g (3 oz), kipper (baked) 21 µg per 85 g (3 oz), salmon (canned) 12 µg per 100 g (3^1/$_2$ oz), sardines (canned) 7.5 µg per 100 g (3^1/$_2$ oz), pilchards (canned) 4.5 µg per 55 g (2 oz), tuna (canned) 2.5 µg per 45 g (1^1/$_2$ oz), risotto (plain) 2 µg per 250 g (9 oz), scrambled eggs (without milk) 2 µg per 100 g (3^1/$_2$ oz), margarine (all types – fortified by law) 0.8 µg per 10 g (^{1}/$_3$ oz).

~ Hot news on minerals and trace elements ~

During the next few years scientists are going to be announcing lots of new discoveries about minerals such as calcium and iron, and trace elements such as selenium and zinc. But don't worry, future findings won't invalidate Eat for Life Diet, because the foods recommended here are rich in these nutrients.

Calcium – How Much?

More than 90 per cent of bone is laid down during growth, and most of the calcium in the body is in bones and teeth. Bone mass peaks at about age 30 to 40 and thereafter declines. In women this process accelerates at the menopause. The DRV report found no evidence that increasing the amount of calcium eaten reduced bone loss. High doses were not recommended because there is thought to be little benefit in eating extra calcium.

For Dietary Reference Values for calcium see Appendix 2

Top ten sources of calcium per portion

Calcium is expressed as milligrams (mg). The food is fresh and raw unless stated otherwise. Where cooked, no sugar is added. Juices are unsweetened. The amounts given are standard portions.

Sprats (fried with bones) 1,364 mg per 220 g ($7^3/_4$ oz), (other fish cooked or canned with bones also good), spinach (boiled) 540 mg per 90 g ($3^1/_4$ oz), cheese and tomato pizza 532 mg per 280 g (10 oz), cheese omelette 420 mg per 150 g ($5^1/_4$ oz), cheese (Cheddar type) 300 mg per 40 g ($1^1/_2$ oz), whole-milk yogurt 300 mg per 150 g ($5^1/_4$ oz), low fat-yogurt 285 mg per 150 g ($5^1/_4$ oz), calcium-fortified milk 262 mg per 40 g ($1^1/_2$ oz), milk pudding (with skimmed milk) 262 mg per 200 g (7 oz), porridge (with milk) 216 mg per 180 g ($6^1/_2$ oz), custard (skimmed milk) 210 mg per 150 g ($5^1/_4$ oz).

Iron – How Much?

Iron is essential for red blood cells and most is recycled by the body, although some is lost through bleeding. Those most at risk of anaemia (shortage of haemoglobin, the oxygen-carrying pigment of the red blood cells,) are adolescents and menstruating women. The DRV panel had difficulty setting levels because iron of animal origin is absorbed more efficiently than iron from vegetable sources, although vitamin C helps this. Other factors in the diet can also inhibit absorption, such as tannin in tea. The EAR set in the DRVs will cover the needs of 75 per cent of women, with the RNI covering 90 per cent. About 10 per cent of women may need iron tablets. Pregnant women with low iron stores may need tablets, too, but normal healthy mothers do not need extra iron, as menstrual loss will not be adding to their needs.

For Dietary Reference Values for iron see Appendix 2

Top ten sources of iron per portion

Iron is expressed as milligrams (mg). The food is fresh and raw unless stated otherwise. Where cooked, no sugar is added. Juices are unsweetened. The amounts given are standard portions.

Liver (pig, stewed) 24 mg per 142 g (5 oz) (and other offal), breakfast cereals such as Sultana Bran 17 per mg 40 g ($1^{1}/_{2}$ oz), sprats (fried) 8.5 mg per 190 g ($6^{3}/_{4}$ oz), cockles (boiled) 6.5 mg per 25 g (scant 1 oz) (and other shellfish), chicken curry (without bones) 5.5 mg per 300 g (11 oz), bulghur wheat 5 mg per 100 g ($3^{1}/_{2}$ oz), sardines (canned) 4.5 mg per 100 g ($3^{1}/_{2}$ oz) (and other oily fish canned or cooked with bones), cauliflower bhajia 4 mg per 140 g (5 oz), bread such as wholemeal pitta 2.5 mg per 95 g ($3^{1}/_{4}$ oz).

Zinc – How Much?

Zinc is vital for several enzyme systems and for building cells. The body is quite good at conserving zinc. Absorption increases in pregnancy so there is no extra requirement. Too much zinc (2 g) produces nausea and vomiting, and long-term high intakes interfere with the absorption of other minerals.

For Dietary Reference Values for zinc see Appendix 2

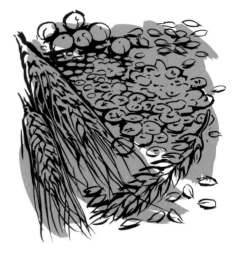

Top ten sources of zinc per portion

Zinc is expressed as milligrams (mg). The food is fresh and raw unless stated otherwise. Where cooked, no sugar is added. Juices are unsweetened. The amounts given are standard portions.

Liver (pig, stewed) 11 mg per 142 g (5 oz) (and other types of liver), breakfast cereals such as Start 7.5 mg per 40 g ($1^{1}/_{2}$ oz), lamb (breast, lean only) 6 mg per 120 g ($4^{1}/_{4}$ oz) (and other types of lamb), beef rump steak (grilled lean only) 6 mg per 142 g (5 oz) (and other types of beef), gammon rashers (grilled, lean only) 6 mg per 170 g (6 oz), oysters 4.5 mg per 170 g (6 oz), pork chops, loin (grilled, lean only) 3.5 mg per 100 g ($3^{1}/_{2}$ oz), shrimps (boiled) 3 mg per 60 g ($2^{1}/_{4}$ oz), turkey (roast, dark meat) 3 mg per 90 g ($3^{1}/_{4}$ oz), ox heart (stewed) 3 mg per 85 g (3 oz), sardines (canned) 3 mg per 100 g ($3^{1}/_{2}$ oz).

Potassium – How Much?

Potassium helps balance sodium and the fluid within the cells, and it enables nerves and muscles to function. To avoid high blood pressure the DRV panel advises taking enough potassium to enable sodium to be excreted. However, they could not establish a recommended amount.

For Dietary Reference Values for potassium see Appendix 2

Top ten sources of potassium per portion

Potassium is expressed as milligrams (mg). The food is fresh and raw unless stated otherwise. Where cooked, no sugar is added. Juices are unsweetened. The amounts given are standard portions.
Mixed vegetable curry 1,248 mg per 300 g (11 oz), green plantain (fried) 1,220 mg per 200 g (7 oz), old potatoes (baked) 1088 mg per 160 g (5³/₄ oz), herring curry 1,047 mg per 300 g (11 oz) (and other types of oily fish), dried apricots (stewed) 600 mg per 85g (3 oz), pomegranate 583 mg per 154 g (5¹/₂ oz), rhubarb (stewed) 560 mg per 140 g (5 oz), tomato juice 494 mg per 190 g (6³/₄ oz), cantaloupe melon 480 mg per 150 g (5¹/₄ oz), kedgeree 480 mg per 300 g (11 oz).

Selenium – How Much?

Selenium is part of an enzyme that helps prevent damage from free radicals. The amount of enzyme produced increases, up to a point, with selenium intake. However, the DRV panel felt that insufficient information was available to set EARs. As too much selenium can be harmful an upper intake is 6 µg per kilogram (2¹/₄ lb) weight a day for adults.

For Dietary Reference Values for selenium see Appendix 2

Good sources of selenium per portion

Levels vary widely, depending on the soil in which the crop has been grown or where the animals for meat and milk have been grazing. Selenium is expressed as micrograms µg. Food fresh and raw unless stated otherwise. Where cooked, no sugar added. Juices unsweetened. The amount given are standard portions.
Liver (grilled) 56 µg per 140 g (5 oz), white fish (grilled) 38 µg per 120 g (4¹/₄ oz), lamb (roast) 25 µg per 140 g (5 oz), brown rice

18 µg per 150 g (5^1/$_2$ oz), prawns (shelled) 13 µg per 40 g (1^1/$_2$ oz), museli (brown crunchy) 10 µg per 80 g (3 oz), milk 1.5 µg to 15 µg per 300 ml (^{1}/$_2$ pint), eggs 3 µg to 28 µg per size 3 egg.

~ Should you keep taking the pills? ~

Although we need vitamins and minerals on a daily basis, the received advice is that, with a few exceptions such as a woman's iron needs in pregnancy, nutrients should be obtained from food and not as dietary supplements.

One reason for caution about vitamin and mineral pills is that vitamins probably act together with other substances in food, such as fibre, minerals and possibly some as-yet unknown substances. These additional ingredients are unlikely to be in vitamin pills.

Taking vitamin and mineral pills can also upset the natural balance. For example, in food the B vitamins are invariably found in clusters, so taking B vitamins individually as vitamin supplements may upset some body processes, or create additional requirements. This might be as harmful as not eating enough vitamins. All the more reason to eat well.

Scientific trials in America are trying to discover whether we do get enough ACE nutrients from food. 'Intervention' trials, in which some people are put on a course of antioxidant vitamin tablets, while others are given placebo (dummy) tablets, are underway by the National Cancer Institute of the National Institutes of Health.

The levels of vitamins being given are above the Recommended Dietary Allowances recognised by the American government as necessary to prevent deficiency diseases. That in itself indicates that scientists suspect higher levels are needed to protect against heart disease and cancer. However, it may not be the case, and until we know the results the advice remains to take your vitamins and minerals in the form of foods.

IN THE BALANCE

If you eat more fruit and veg are you increasing your intake of pesticide residues? Probably. Not everyone can afford – or find – organically grown fruit and vegetables. At any rate, not all organic produce is free from residues. That is not to say that producers are cheating, but even though a system of agriculture may have no chemical input, it can still be contaminated.

While the debate about pesticide residues rages, the conclusion of the scientific experts is that any potential risk from residues is outweighed by the benefit of the expected reduction in chronic diseases attributed to eating more fruit, vegetable and starchy CC foods. Avoiding eating fruit and vegetables would result in a diet of fatty, sugary foods – which would quickly lead to weight problems and in the long-term could produce more serious problems.

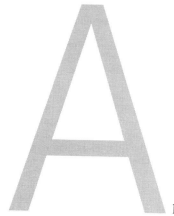

The Preventive Powers of ACE Eating

A healthy diet containing plenty of vitamins and minerals is essential for preventing certain diseases. Based on the latest nutritional findings, Eat for Life Diet is built round 'ACE eating' – eating foods rich in beta carotene (for vitamin A) and vitamins C and E – along with other nutrient-dense 'superfoods'. It is no exaggeration to call it the 'healthiest diet in the world'. Scientists believe that both superfoods and supernutrients help protect against a variety of diseases and health problems.

~ *Protecting against coronary heart disease* ~

The UK has one of the highest rates of heart disease in the world and other north and central European countries are not far behind. Some of the causes of heart disease that you can do something about are smoking, lack of exercise and an unhealthy diet.

One of the main causes of heart disease is high levels of blood cholesterol. Usually the body maintains a balance of blood cholesterol, making more if needed and excreting excess. But eating too much saturated fat can raise blood cholesterol levels.

There are two main types of blood cholesterol. The 'good' type is high density lipoprotein (HDL) which carries excess cholesterol to the liver for removal from the body. The 'bad' type is low density lipoprotein (LDL) which deposits cholesterol in the artery walls. Adequate amounts of HDL are associated with a lower risk of heart disease. Eating a diet high in fat, especially saturated fat, but not necessarily dietary cholesterol increases the amount of LDL.

Attempts at reducing fat intake in the UK haven't focussed on dietary cholesterol because the amount of cholesterol eaten does not usually raise blood cholesterol as much as saturated fat does. However, the World Health Organisation (WHO) considers the

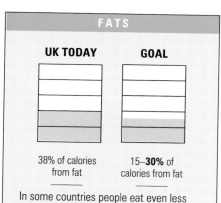

FATS

UK TODAY	GOAL
38% of calories from fat	15–**30%** of calories from fat

In some countries people eat even less than 30 per cent of their calories as fat, but this amount would mean that the British diet would have to change drastically, so 30 per cent is a realistic target for the present. WHO thinks further benefits might be expected in the future by aiming for a fat intake approaching 15 per cent of total calories.

amount of cholesterol eaten to be important and has set a limit of 300 mg per day on dietary cholesterol because there is some evidence that high intakes are linked with an increased risk of heart disease.

The body can make all the cholesterol it needs, so none has to be eaten. Dietary cholesterol is found only in animal foods; the richest sources are liver, shellfish and eggs. High levels are also found in fatty meats, high-fat cheese and full-fat milk, but as these foods are also high in saturated fat they should be limited anyway. They don't have to be given up completely; just try not to eat them too regularly.

The British view on cholesterol is that it is more practical to concentrate on lowering total fat and saturated fat intakes. This has a more direct effect on blood cholesterol levels than avoiding cholesterol-containing foods does. Meeting Eat for Life Diet goals for saturated fat will help take care of cholesterol.

Reports that low cholesterol levels put people at increased risk of cancer have been dismissed. Low cholesterol levels are probably a result of the cancer – not a cause or a risk factor.

Polyunsaturated fats have been shown to help reduce blood cholesterol levels, and the Eat for Life lower limit of 3 per cent of total calories ensures you have enough of the essential fatty acids which the body cannot make but which are needed for essential growth and maintenance. The upper limit is 7 per cent, but there is no actual need to eat more than 3 per cent, although the DRV report specifies an upper limit of 10 per cent.

There is an upper limit on polyunsaturates because studies on animals suggest that excessive intake might increase the risk of certain cancers, although there is no evidence that polyunsaturates have been associated with human disease. Where laboratory experiments have suggested that polyunsatuates are implicated in cancer, it is at levels far above anything eaten in a normal diet. It's likely that if there are problems they are linked to existing disease and are not actually causing disease.

In the world's healthiest diets polyunsaturate intake rarely goes above 10 per cent. As no disease has been associated with intakes at that level – and no benefits are known for higher intakes – this has been set as the safe upper limit.

The high intakes of monounsaturates in Mediterranean

SATURATED FATS

UK TODAY	GOAL

16% of calories from saturated fat

No more than 10% of calories from saturated fat

Eating too much saturated fat can raise cholesterol levels and can increase our risk of heart disease.

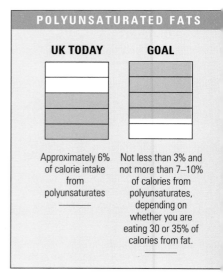

POLYUNSATURATED FATS

UK TODAY	GOAL

Approximately 6% of calorie intake from polyunsaturates

Not less than 3% and not more than 7–10% of calories from polyunsaturates, depending on whether you are eating 30 or 35% of calories from fat.

CC POWER vs HEART DISEASE

Diets high in CC foods are usually associated with fewer heart attacks. The reason could be that meeting the Eat for Life Diet goal of CC foods contributing at least half of total calories just doesn't leave room for a substantial intake of foods high in saturated fats.

countries, such as olive oil and rapeseed oil, have been suggested as a reason for low rates of heart disease. The expert view is that where low rates occur it is more likely due to a low intake of saturated fats. So far, there's not enough evidence to say that monounsaturates can help prevent heart disease. Therefore there is no Eat for Life Diet goal for monounsaturates.

However, there's no reason to reduce our current intake of 12 per cent of calories from monounsaturates. Both the WHO scientists and the British DRV experts are happy for mono-unsaturates to make up the difference between the total fat intake and the sum of the saturated and polyunsaturated fats: in other words, 12–13 per cent of total calories can come from monounsaturates.

~ *Protecting against cancer* ~

It is estimated that 85 per cent of cancers may be avoidable and can be attributed to diet, smoking, drinking alcohol, excessive exposure to sun and pollution. Of that total, 35 per cent of all cancer deaths have been estimated to be related to diet.

A high intake of fat, and of saturated fat in particular, is associated with an increased risk of cancers of the breast, colon and prostate. Achieving the Eat for Life Diet goals for fats and polyunsaturates (see pages 43–44) should go some way to reducing these risks, but WHO has predicted that fat intake may have to be reduced even further in future as more evidence on fat and cancer becomes available.

Diets rich in green and yellow vegetables and citrus fruit are associated with a lower incidence of some cancers. Low levels of beta carotene in the blood have also been noted among people who have cancer, but this may be a result of the cancer, rather than a cause. Some scientists also think low levels of vitamin E coupled with low levels of selenium and vitamin C may also indicate a risk. Although it is not fully understood why this could be so, there is data showing that fruit and vegetables play a protective role in preventing certain cancers, probably more due to beta carotene than vitamin A; but it could be due to other factors.

Even though more evidence is needed, scientists are confident enough to say that a diet low in total and saturated fat; high in plant food (especially green and yellow vegetables and citrus fruit); low in alcohol, and low in salt-pickled, smoked and salt-preserved foods will help prevent many of the major cancers in the world today. And it certainly won't harm anyone.

~ *Protecting against osteoporosis* ~

Osteoporosis, in which bones lose their density and become fragile, is a common problem. Half of all women suffer a hip fracture by the time they are 70. As we are living longer today, it is something to be aware of, especially as diet and exercise earlier in life can help prevent the problem.

Bone mass peaks around the age of 30 to 40 then begins to decline. The decline accelerates at the menopause and in men from the age of about 55. If your bone density is high in mid-life you probably won't become osteoporotic. Osteoporosis, like heart disease, has many causes, including insufficient exercise, smoking, excessive alcohol intake, insufficient oestrogen (a female hormone), low calcium intake and possibly some drug therapies. Too much protein and too much salt in the diet can increase calcium loss from the bones.

Adequate calcium intake is important throughout life, particularly during the first six months and around puberty. Even when growth has stopped it is important to maintain calcium intake to ensure maximum mineralisation of the bones by the age of 30, especially for women.

Exercise promotes bone growth and density. During convalescence from illness or accidents that inactivate people, there is calcium loss from the bones which needs to be replaced. For details of calcium rich foods, see page 39.

~ *Protecting against high blood pressure* ~

The risk of a heart attack or a stroke increases with high blood pressure. The first actions to take to help lower blood pressure are losing weight, if necessary, and reducing the amount of alcohol drunk, if necessary,

Under pressure and stress, blood pressure rises, so finding ways of avoiding or reducing stress is another way of lowering blood pressure.

CC POWER vs CANCER

Diets rich in starchy food have consistently been linked with a lower incidence of several cancers. It is probably the combined antioxidant effect of vitamin C and beta carotene (see page 00), together with the fact that these diets are high in CC power, other vitamins, minerals and fibre, that makes them so healthy.

EC CODE ON PREVENTING CANCER

1 Smoking is the greatest risk factor of all. If you smoke, stop as quickly as possible.
2 Go easy on the alcohol. Drinking too much as been linked to 3 per cent of cancers.
3 Avoid being overweight. Some cancers are associated with obesity.
4 Take care in the sun. Too much sun can cause skin cancer.
5 Observe the health and safety regulations at work.
6 Cut down on fatty foods. In Western countries, where people usually eat lot of meat, butter and other dairy products, there is a higher risk of breast and bowel cancer as well as heart disease.
7 Eat plenty of fresh fruit and vegetables and other foods containing fibre.
8 See your doctor if there is any unexplained change in your normal health which lasts for more than two weeks.
And for women...
9 Have a regular cervical smear test.
10 Examine your breasts monthly.

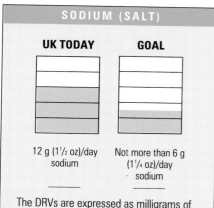

SODIUM (SALT)

UK TODAY	GOAL
12 g (1½ oz)/day sodium	Not more than 6 g (1¼ oz)/day sodium

The DRVs are expressed as milligrams of sodium, a component of salt. The DRV panel says only a fraction of the sodium eaten is needed. Lowering sodium intake could be of benefit in reducing high blood pressure and heart disease, especially as there is a relationship between sodium intake and rise in blood pressure as you get older. Although no EARs for sodium were set, lower and upper intakes have been set. For Dietary Reference Values for sodium see Appendix 2.

Doctors should also advise people with high blood pressure to reduce salt intake, since salt and high blood pressure are linked (though whether salt causes the problem is still controversial). The Eat for Life Diet goal of not more than 6 g (1/4 oz) per day – half the amount eaten now – includes both salt added at the table and salt already in cooked and processed foods.

Hard exercise and exposure to high temperatures, which cause the body to sweat heavily, may create a need for more sodium in the short-term. However, the body will adapt to the new conditions, which rules out a long-term need for extra sodium – and any excuses about not cutting down!

Other minerals such as potassium and magnesium, which are abundant in CC foods, fruit and vegetables, are important because they probably have a balancing effect on sodium, helping to limit rises in blood pressure. (For more information about potassium, see page 41. For DRVS see Appendix 2.)

Reducing fat intake is also beneficial because it is the food most likely to result in weight gain, and being overweight contributes to high blood pressure.

~ Protecting against stress ~

Stress is linked with high blood pressure and ultimately heart disease. The secret of success over stress is to recognise the events that trigger stress and to learn to use anti-stress techniques such as deep breathing or whatever works for you. Tell-tale signs of stress include:

- being irritable and depressed
- lack of concentration
- inability to make decisions
- difficulty in sleeping
- turning more often to drink or cigarettes.

Even though it's popularly thought that smoking and alcohol are 'relaxing', in fact they are stimulants that put the body under more stress and leave you more tired. Alcohol and cigarettes also impair absorption of B vitamins and increase the need for vitamin C.

Controlling alcohol intake and taking up exercise are two other strategies for alleviating stress. Exercise has a relaxing effect on the body and is a natural antidote to stress (even though it might not seem like it at the time) because it triggers the release of endorphins in the brain – natural pain-killers that produce a sense of well-being, or the 'high' familiar to those who exercise.

Whether stress per se increases the body's need for vitamins and minerals, especially the B vitamins and vitamin C is debatable. Either way Eat for Life Diet supplies valuable nutrients, and acts as a reminder of the importance to eat well; easily forgotten at times of stress.

~ *Protecting against gallstones* ~

Gallstones are formed by blood cholesterol and bile and are more common among people eating only limited amounts of fruit, vegetables, bread and cereals. Those most likely to have gallstones are fair, fat, over 40 and female although other people may also have them. The good news is that you can change the composition of bile to make it less likely to form stones by altering your diet to include lots of CC foods.

~ *Protecting some diabetics* ~

Maturity-onset diabetes, the kind of diabetes that comes on later in life, is associated with an increased risk of heart disease and other health problems. Being obese is one of the major risk factors in this non-insulin-dependent diabetes. About 80 per cent of sufferers are obese. Fortunately, this kind of diabetes can usually be reversed or at least managed more easily by losing weight and taking exercise.

Virtually all diabetics, both those with insulin-dependence, and those with non-insulin-dependent diabetes, are now advised to eat lots of CC foods, fruit and vegetables and to go easy on fat, particularly saturated fat – the pattern of eating in the Eat for Life Diet.

~ *Protecting against dental caries* ~

Toothbrush and toothpaste are excellent weapons against plaque and gum disease, but food also has a fundamental effect. Free sugars are known to be responsible for tooth decay, or dental caries (holes in the teeth). Eat for Life Diet goals include an upper limit on these destructive free sugars.

Of course, as an individual you will inherit 'good' or 'bad' teeth, or rather their susceptibility to decay, but there is also a direct relationship between the frequency with which sugar is eaten and the number of caries in the teeth. Crudely, the more often you eat sugar, the more drilling and filling you will need. (See also page 56.)

~ *Protecting against anaemia* ~

Anaemia is a potential problem for lots of women, especially those on crash diets that don't include nutrient-dense Eat for Life Diet superfoods, and for infants and teenagers whose diets don't measure up to these standards!

The protective powers of fruit and vegetables are extensive. Because they contribute a lot of vitamin C, they can improve iron status. Whereas the iron in animal foods is easily absorbed by the body, the iron in vegetable foods needs vitamin C to convert it for use. (See page 20.) Achieving the Eat for Life Diet's goal of five portions a day of fruit and vegetables will therefore help prevent anaemia. CC foods also give added protection because wholegrain foods are richer in iron.

~ *Protecting against cataracts* ~

Cataracts are the single biggest cause of blindness in the world and a common problem among the elderly in Britain. ACE eating may also help prevent cataracts. The evidence is far from conclusive, but why wait when improving your diet cannot do any harm and will have so many other benefits?

Some cataracts may be caused by oxidation of the lens in the eye, and antioxidant vitamins like C and E and beta carotene may help prevent this. It has been estimated by some medical researchers that people with low vitamin C and low carotenoid levels are many times more likely to develop cataracts. Vitamin E has been less strongly associated with cataracts in this initial research.

~ *Protecting against pregnancy problems* ~

If you are expecting a baby, or planning a family, the Eat for Life Diet's revelations apply especially to you. By about the end of the first month of pregnancy (often before many women realise they are expecting a baby) most of the embryo's basic formation is nearing completion. Nutrient-rich superfoods and ACE eating are therefore especially important early on – ideally, prior to conception. An increased intake of foods high in folic acid before conception is particularly advisable (see page 37).

Eating well at all times is the best strategy for women. This prevents the need for a sudden change in diet at a time when you might be suffering morning sickness, or food cravings. And during pregnancy slimming is not advised, unless under medical supervision. Being in shape before becoming pregnant makes weight loss easier after the birth.

There is no need to 'eat for two' during pregnancy. In fact, you only need an extra 200 calories a day, during the third trimester (after 28 weeks). But make sure those calories are well 'spent' on superfoods such as low-fat milk, yogurt and CC foods, as they offer a growing baby lots of nutrients.

Nutrient-dense foods can also play a vital role towards the end of pregnancy, when normal-sized meals might cause indigestion. Snacking on superfoods might be easier.

In general, throughout pregnancy eat lots of starchy food, lots of fruit and vegetables, and one lean protein meal a day.

~ Protecting against ageing ~

Diet matters at any age, but when you become less active you will need fewer calories so it is wise to make the most of them with nutrient-dense foods to protect health and prevent weight problems.

For the older person who lives alone, there may be less motivation for meal planning. And when absorption of vitamins and minerals may be impaired by aging, or by various drugs and medication, it's especially important to safeguard nutritional quality. Including as many CC foods as possible also prevents constipation.

If false teeth mean it is impossible to bite into fresh fruit, cut it up and chew well because chewing stimulates saliva (and appetite) and it brings out the taste. Stew fresh or dried fruit, drink fruit juices, and eat lots of cooked vegetables. Protein needs should take care of themselves if calorie intake is enough, but lean meat and fish are still best.

Finally, no lesser authority than the Royal College of Physicians says exercising into old age helps keep you physically young. It also helps to prevent heart disease, post-menopausal osteoporosis, maturity-onset diabetes, and bone and joint problems.

The Junior Eat for Life Diet

Healthy eating should start young. When they are growing, children need plenty of energy and nutrient-dense foods. And because there is mounting evidence that diseases of adult life might have their roots in childhood diet and lifestyle, it's all the more important to pay attention to early diet.

The process of atherosclerosis (narrowing and furring up of the arteries) which leads to heart disease, starts in childhood and is strongly linked to a diet rich in saturated fat and low in CC foods (complex carbohydrates). That does not mean that children ought to be put on faddy diets that are too low in fat and/or too high in fibre, which might sometimes lead to rare incidents of 'muesli belt malnutrition' that make the headlines. After all, children have small stomachs and large energy needs, so their meals need to be more frequent and more regular than adults.

~ Weaning little ones ~

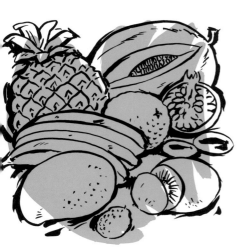

Weaning babies off their milk diet – and all reports agree that breast is best – happens at different ages for different babies although solids shouldn't be introduced before three months.

Whenever it happens, a baby must not be weaned on to a high-fibre, low-fat diet immediately. Even after weaning, babies derive a lot of nutrients and energy from milk. First solid foods should be purées of vegetables and some fruit (not berries, which can cause allergic reactions). The emphasis is on fresh foods, although the occasional jar, can or packet of babyfood is not harmful.

Purées can gradually become thicker and incorporate baby cereals such as rice until the baby is eating food mashed with a fork. By six months of age the baby should be having a balanced diet with a little meat, fish or beans and pulses, some milk or yogurt, cereals, fruit and vegetables. Egg, cow's milk and wheat cereals should not be introduced before this age, in case they provoke an allergy or intolerance.

~ Milky way ~

After weaning, babies may require full-fat milk until they are two, when they can switch to semi-skimmed. From the age of two the advice is usually to keep to semi-skimmed rather than skimmed, but if you are confident that your two-year-old is obtaining enough calories from other foods, skimmed could be introduced earlier. After all, toddlers can be perfectly healthy without cow's milk – some are allergic to it – but it is a convenient source of calories. Of course, the question of whether to choose low-fat or semi-skimmed milk becomes rather academic if crisps, chocolates and other sources of saturated fat are regularly eaten!

~ Fat-finding ~

While it is very tempting to give in to what children 'like' (or what advertisers, motorway cafés and fast-food restaurants tell us they like), in general the emphasis (as with adults) should be on fat contributing only a modest amount of energy in a child's diet, with more unsaturated fat than saturated. Controlling the amount of fat a child eats will help control his or her weight.

Fat provides few vitamins, but children need some for their bodies to grow and function properly. Of all age groups, theirs is the one that can eat most energy-dense foods. If all their food is bulky and low-calorie, very young children may simply be unable to eat enough to meet their needs. However, there obviously needs to be a balance, because a government survey of British schoolchildren's eating habits shows that three-quarters of children are getting more than 35 per cent of their calories from fat – mainly from chips, burgers and biscuits. The Eat for Life Diet goal of about 30 per cent is safe for children.

Most of our lifelong eating habits are formed in childhood, so learning the Eat for Life Diet habit early on means it will be easier to stay slim and healthy. Too often we associate fatty and sugary

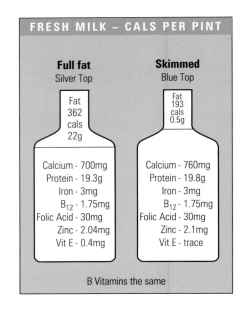

FRESH MILK – CALS PER PINT

Full fat Silver Top	**Skimmed** Blue Top
Fat 362 cals 22g	Fat 193 cals 0.5g
Calcium - 700mg	Calcium - 760mg
Protein - 19.3g	Protein - 19.8g
Iron - 3mg	Iron - 3mg
B_{12} - 1.75mg	B_{12} - 1.75mg
Folic Acid - 30mg	Folic Acid - 30mg
Zinc - 2.04mg	Zinc - 2.1mg
Vit E - 0.4mg	Vit E - trace

B Vitamins the same

foods with rewards: sweets, cakes, biscuits are given to children for being 'good'. Vegetables are seen as a punishment food: 'No pudding unless you eat up your greens.' As well as consciously avoiding this approach, involve your child in picking out the fruit and vegetables at the supermarket or greengrocer's, and when they are old enough let them help prepare the vegetables (even though it takes time and is messy).

Remember that you are your child's role-model. They will enjoy the food you enjoy.

It is kinder to form healthy tastes and habits early on, especially as this is the time bodies need lots of nutrients to reach their full physical and mental potential. Changing habits later in life is much, much harder.

~ ACE eating for children ~

There is a need to encourage children to eat foods rich in vitamins A, C and E – the key superfoods in the Eat for Life Diet. Once children go outside the home, they need little encouragement to eat the 'other' type of fatty and sugary food!

Start them off snacking on fruit, raw vegetable sticks, wholemeal sandwiches and toast, dried fruits, thin parings (not great chunks) of cheese, breakfast cereals. And for children over four who are not at risk of choking, nuts (not the salted and roasted varieties, but those mixed with dried fruits). Make these the only accessible snacks in the house, so that children (and adults) reach for them automatically instead of heading straight for the biscuit box. Children who have such habits early on stand a better chance than those with their noses stuck permanently in a crisp bag.

Find out what foods are offered at your child's school and, if necessary, try to influence the food choices. Local authorities are becoming more aware of the importance of healthy school dinners, and many maintain strict nutritional controls over school meals. For example, a school may offer chips only once a week and perhaps have a 'healthy-food' tuck shop. However, authorities do vary, and some still operate the 'cafeteria' system where a child can choose chips and chocolate every day if he or she wishes.

~ Get up and go ~

Diet alone won't protect children from ill health later in life. Exercise has to be a part of their lifestyle to build strong bones and muscles so they reach their full potential. Aerobic exercise is as important for the young as it is for the old. And a new report by the Royal College of Physicians, *Medical Aspects of Exercise: Risks and Benefits*, concludes that the habit of exercise is best started in childhood – and continued through middle-age into old age. Their findings are that exercise protects against heart disease, osteoporosis and other ills. They also say less than one-fifth of children take enough exercise to maintain or improve health.

To make it fun for children means finding something that suits a child's personality, from walking (or running) the family dog, to abseiling. Some children will enjoy team sports and some will prefer testing themselves in individual activities. Some will need cajoling – even bribing – but once the habit is established it becomes easier.

~ What if the children go vegetarian? ~

If children reject animal products, for whatever reason, and decide to go vegetarian – don't panic! The Eat For Life Diet's principles and Eating Plans offer vegetarian alternatives. Another way is to increase the number of vegetarian days in the rest of the family's eating to make catering easier.

So long as a 'veggiemite' is eating enough calories from a well-balanced selection of vegetarian foods, including cereals and grains, nuts, seeds and pulses, then there is nothing to worry about in terms of protein.

Don't worry that children who don't eat meat won't grow – it's not true. There are plenty of vegetarians who row, climb mountains or run marathons, and plenty of others who are academics.

~ Start pumping iron ~

As there is some evidence that anaemia occurs in Western society among young children (and pregnant women and the elderly), iron is another important consideration for all children, but especially

GOING OFF FOOD

When children go off food, it is usually because they are sickening for one of the 'routine' illnesses of childhood, from sniffles to measles. A sick child uses its energy for fighting the disease – not digesting food. It is quite natural in these circumstances to 'go off' food, and nothing to worry about.

Like adults, children automatically adjust the amount they eat to meet their energy needs. This happens subconsciously over a period of days to compensate for over- and under-eating. However, if a child does not eat for more than a couple of days, call the doctor. When they go off meals, they might eat small snacks. If they have diarrhoea, you must make sure they drink plenty of fluids, or give replacement salts if necessary – consult your GP.

With a genuinely faddy eater, it may be advisable to seek help from a dietitian or your doctor or health visitor.

vegetarian children. In animal foods iron occurs in the haem form. This is used more easily by the body than the non-haem form, which occurs in plant foods such as dark green vegetables, dried fruit, nuts, whole grains, soya flour, oatmeal, wholemeal bread and flour. Eating foods rich in vitamin C along with plant sources of iron is necessary to enhance its absorption. This happens naturally in the food recommendations in the Eat for Life Diet.

Zinc also comes mainly from meat and like iron is more readily absorbed by the body when it comes from animal sources. Vegetarian sources of zinc are brewer's yeast, cheese, eggs, carrots, peanuts, green beans, tomatoes, peas, potatoes, sweetcorn, whole grain cereals such as brown rice and wholemeal bread and breakfast cereals. As with iron, the body makes the best use of zinc when it is taken with foods rich in vitamin C.

~ And if children go vegan...? ~

A vegan diet for growing children is much more restrictive and therefore needs to be done with care. Without vitamin B12 there is a risk of anaemia. Those who don't eat animal products often obtain less B12 than they need. However, the folic acid that is needed to work with vitamin B12 is in plentiful supply in a good vegan diet. Foods supplemented with B12, such as yeast extract, some breakfast cereals and soya products, are necessary for vegan children (and adults).

Feeding a vegan also needs particular attention to calcium. There is plenty in dairy foods but, for those who don't eat them, calcium is found in the following: cereals, muesli, oatmeal, beans, pulses, nuts, seeds, dark green vegetables, dried fruit especially figs, white bread, soya milk and soya milk 'yogurt' and desserts.

~ Teething problems ~

The Junior Eat for Life Diet also gives children something to smile about later in life, since diet affects teeth in two ways. First, a good diet is essential even when babies are toothless because minerals are needed to form teeth before they erupt. This means that breastfeeding mums and young infants need to eat a good diet. Later on, when the second teeth are formed, diet is also important.

Second, once teeth have erupted, food has a direct effect on them. Eat for Life Diet provides the nutrients needed to form healthy teeth and bones.

Different foods may increase or decrease the size and number of dental caries. Despite the rumours you may have heard to the contrary, eating apples and other fruit does not increase the number of fillings children (and adults) will need. Fruit does contain sugars, but they are not as bad for teeth as sweets and sugar are. Although fruit juices can wear enamel off the teeth, they do contain vitamins and minerals. It's best to dilute fruit juices for children – which saves money, as well as teeth. Of course, if you add sugar to cooked fruit that does increase the risk of dental caries.

The lactose (milk sugar) in milk is not harmful to teeth either. Some people have said that starchy foods give you dental caries, but the bulk of evidence shows that starchy foods like bread and potatoes, rice and pasta are not a problem.

Very few caries occur when consumption of free sugar is less than 30 g (1 oz) a day. A steep increase occurs at 60 g (2 1/4 oz) a day. The more often sugar and sugary foods are put in the mouth, the more likely people are to get caries. Sucking sweets and chewing toffees and eating sugary snacks between meals spells teething trouble.

~ Takeaway tactics for teenagers ~

Adolescents, for whatever reason, are less likely to eat what, when and where you choose. If they are determined to live on junk food as a way of rebelling, there's not a lot you can do. Try appealing to their concern for the environment or animal welfare – or their vanity. To look good they'd be well advised to revise their eating habits, or make some 'educated' choices of takeaways.

There are several approaches here. Persuade them to bring the takeaway home to eat (or have it delivered) then you can offer home-made, low-fat milk shakes, plain milk or fruit juice, either on its own or mixed with fizzy water, instead of the takeaway's drinks laden with sugar, artificial sweetener and colouring. However, the occasional cola isn't harmful. At home you can also supply additional salad without the fatty dressing. Baked potatoes

---

CHILDREN'S PARTIES

If the principles of Eat for Life Diet form the basis of children's eating habits, then the occasional party meal of 'jelly and ice-cream', or whatever is the latest craze in savoury snacks or sticky confectionery bars, won't do any harm. Socialising is more important than sticking rigidly to nutrition principles which could make food an issue and a barrier between parents, children and their friends.

However, there is no need to go to the other extreme just to comply with current party conventions. Make your own conventions. If the food is colourful and presented in fun, fanciful ways, even children who are used to sausage rolls and fairy cakes at parties may not notice that the food is good for them!

or bread can be provided as substitutes for the fries, or you could produce the occasional batch of home-made thick-cut chips and fry them in polyunsaturated oil.

Encourage them to make burgers only occasional meals – and definitely not snacks. A burger may appear to be small, but with all the fatty trimmings of processed cheese and mayonnaise it supplies about half a teenage girl's daily calorie requirements.

Suggest grilled rather than fried fast foods and thicker-cut chips, oven-cooked if possible; also, avoid those chip shops that reheat by double-frying. Suggest foods without batter, which soaks up more fat. Choose whole pieces of fish or meat rather than 'nuggets', which give less meat and expose even more batter and surfaces to soak up fat. Explain that 'extra crisp' usually indicates extra fat has been added for crisping.

Don't worry if children are pizza freaks – at least pizzas contain more nutrients than confectionery! Suggest some vegetarian pizza toppings and pizzas without cheese or meat, as they are lower in fat. Deep pan pizzas offer more base which means more starchy bread to counteract any fatty sausage or salami.

~ Hollow-leg syndrome ~

Growing youngsters who are always hungry can be satisfied quickly and relatively cheaply with the Eat for Life Diet's CC foods. Fill them up with bread, rice, pasta or potatoes, as well as lots of vegetables at every meal, with fruit as snacks. And let them eat cake – wholemeal ones such as fruit, date and walnut, carrot, malt loaf, teacake, Hot Cross buns, scones. These are all good low fat bakes (so long as they are not spread with lashings of butter or icing). In general, provide a wide variety of foods and try to confiscate the sugar bowl.

~ Leaving home ~

As teenagers increasingly make their own decisions about food, and will soon be completely independent, arm them with the basic information (such as a copy of the Eat for Life Diet) so they can select a healthy diet for themselves.

An illustration such as the healthy-eating pyramid shows graphically that the foundation of a healthy diet is CC food, on which are built the five-portions-a-day of fruit and vegetables. The rest is made up from vegetarian foods or lean meat, fish or low fat dairy produce. Drinks aren't shown, but the advice is to quench your thirst on plenty of water, then drink fruit juices and skimmed milk, if milk is liked as a drink. Go easy on caffeine containing drinks such as coffee, tea, cola – find some herb or fruit tea alternatives that you like. Adolescents should also watch their alcohol intake – see pages 86–88 for 'safe' drinking limits.

The Eat for Life Diet is not an expensive way to eat, but before teenagers leave home some guidance or practice in budgeting would be a good idea. Get older teenagers to budget for the family for a week and do the shopping. Offer to teach them a few cooking techniques, and familiarise with good cheap foods: pasta, pulses, root vegetables, cabbage, offal, canned tomatoes, oily fish such as herring and mackerel, rice and bread (see pages 97–146 for recipes).

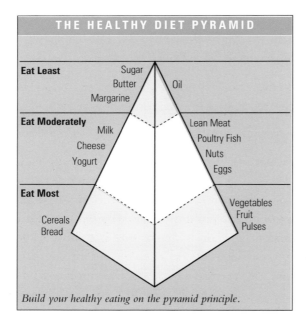

THE HEALTHY DIET PYRAMID

Eat Least — Sugar, Butter, Margarine, Oil

Eat Moderately — Milk, Cheese, Yogurt, Lean Meat, Poultry Fish, Nuts, Eggs

Eat Most — Cereals, Bread, Vegetables, Fruit, Pulses

Build your healthy eating on the pyramid principle.

CHAPTER SIX

Lose Weight Once and For All

f you are reading this specifically because you want to lose weight, then we want to help you achieve your ambition within the framework of the Healthiest Diet in the World.

While you probably want to follow the Eat for Life Diet to enhance your appearance, we also want you to do it to improve your health, which is why we have placed the 28-day Slimming Plan here – after you have read the basic principles about healthy eating. You will have gathered by now that adopting these principles will lead to a gradual weight loss for those who have pounds to shed. But if you want to do it slightly more quickly – or you simply like to have the menus and recipes worked out for you – then here is the Eat for Life Diet Slimming Plan.

~ Enjoy eating ~

This is the most positive slimming diet ever. If you stick with the Eat for Life Diet goals of (1) Eating around half your calories as starchy foods such as bread, pasta, cereals and potatoes - without lots of butter or margarine, and (2) eating at least 400 g (14 oz) of fruit and vegetables a day, you will automatically reduce your fat intake (the third goal of the diet) and bring down your weight without going through the agony of constantly restricting yourself.

Eat for Life Diet positively encourages you to eat because it is now understood that on a low-fat diet like this you don't have to go hungry or suffer food cravings. To be slim you have to change the way you eat permanently. So there is absolutely no point going on a crash diet or a slimming diet that you can't live with. Instead Eat for Life Diet shows you how to eat to be slim for life.

~ Slim with CC foods ~

If you skipped Chapter Two, The Healthiest Diet in the World, you will need to know about the unique health attributes of the Eat for Life Diet Slimming Plan.

First, it is based on CC foods. CC is short for complex carbohydrates. These are starchy, fibre-rich foods such as bread, potatoes, pasta, breakfast cereals, grains, beans and pulses. It has now been scientifically proved that these foods are less fattening than fatty foods.

The trouble is, a lot of people confuse CC foods with the 'other' type of carbohydrates – sugar and sugary foods such as cakes and biscuits, which are fattening.

To explain briefly, there are two main types of carbohydrate.

Complex carbohydrates, which are starchy foods such as cereals, bread, pasta, potatoes, pulses and whole grains, and also fruit and vegetables. It's the fibre in CC foods combined with their natural vitamin and mineral content that makes them so valuable to slimmers. This is because many of the effects previously attributed to fibre are now being attributed to different forms of starch in CC foods.

Free sugars is the scientific name for the stuff that has been refined from sugar cane or sugar beet which you buy by the packet, or eat as an ingredient in processed foods, cakes, biscuits and pastries. Free sugars also include honey, glucose syrup, concentrated fruit juices and all the other sugars added when food is processed.

~ Vital discoveries for slimming ~

Three discoveries vital to slimmers have also been made since fibre became news in the 1980s. They help explain why we are now talking about the need to eat more CC foods in order to slim, rather than just adding fibre to foods – which you've heard (and done) before.

1 Fibre alone is not the answer for slimmers. Sprinkling bran on food is no longer good enough. What you have to do to stay slim is eat CC foods that are naturally rich in starch. Eating more of these foods – fruit, vegetables, cereals such as wheat, rice, maize and oats – leaves less room for refined foods that are high in fat and sugar - the dieter's dual enemies. And that is important because we

EAT FOR LIFE DIET – THE MOST TRIED AND TESTED DIET IN THE HISTORY OF THE WORLD

There can be no more natural way of slimming and staying healthy than the Eat for Life Diet, based as it is on the kind of diet that has sustained the human race through 30,000 to 40,000 years of evolution. Although evolution involved adjusting to a diversity of animal and vegetable foods, the diet that brought us to where we are today was based mainly on CC foods, fruit and vegetables, with small amounts of animal foods.

We have only to look at what happens when 'primitive' people uproot and are replanted in the 'civilised' world to know that the Eat for Life Diet makes sense. They become fat, flabby and ill. There are many sad examples, from American Indians to Australian Aborigines. The Aborigines traditionally ate lots of roots and vegetables. During the early 1900s their diet was changed to mostly white-flour foods and sugar. Their lifestyle changed to a sedentary one. How did they fare? High rates of obesity and diabetes, previously unknown, were followed by high blood pressure and heart disease. Don't let it happen to you.

	Hunter-gatherers	Peasant agriculturalists	Modern affluent societies
fat	15–20 g (1/2–2/3 oz)	10–15 g (1/3–1/2 oz)	
sugar		5 g (1/5 oz)	40+ g (1 1/2+ oz)
starch	50–70 g (1 3/4–2 1/2 oz)	60–75 g (2 1/4–2 3/4 oz)	20 g (2/3 oz)
			25–30 g (about 1 oz)
protein	15–20 g (1/2–2/3 oz)	10–15 g (1/3–1/2 oz)	12 g (1/2 oz)
salt (per day)	1 g	5–15 g (1/6–1/2 oz)	10 g (1/3 oz)
fibre (per day)	40 g (1 1/2 oz)	5–15 g (1/6–1/2 oz)	10 g (1/3 oz)

now know that fat is more likely to be turned into body fat than either CC foods or protein are.

2 There have been suggestions that some of the fibres in CC foods is in part resistant to digestion. Of course you obtain calories from the CC foods you eat, but your body may not be able to use all of the calories. To take advantage of the fact that CC foods are lower in calories than other foods, while at the same time being more filling, eat and enjoy.

3 Eating more fruit and vegetables will help you lose weight. Fruit and vegetables are both naturally high in fibre and low in fat – as long as they are not fried or drowned in butter during cooking or serving.

Neither of these two important groups of Eat for Life Diet superfoods – starchy CC foods and fruit and vegetables – are high in free sugars. Scientists worldwide have said we would be better off if we ate a lot less free sugar, which adds to the evidence that following Eat for Life Diet guidelines is an effective method of weight control.

There are other powerful features of the Eat for Life Diet's 28-day Slimming Plan, such as the superfoods (see pages 26–28) that give you the best nutritional value for the lowest calorie cost. Working on the principle that quality is even more important than usual when quantity is reduced, superfoods are a vital ingredient in successful slimming. They also contain the unique combinations of vitamins and minerals – the ACE eating factor (see pages 28–34) – that help protect slimmers against illness and infection.

~ Chubby children ~

Weight problems are becoming more common among school pupils, probably because of a combination of unsuitable diet – too much fatty food – and lack of exercise. Watching television and playing electronic computer games for hours on end, while eating crisps, biscuits and sweets, between burgers, is a sure way to start a weight problem.

Doctors say we need to encourage high levels of physical activity at early ages to help avoid weight problems. If children in your care have weight problems, let them eat the Eat for Life Diet with you. Don't restrict their calorie intake; let them eat as much as they like. The low fat content will help them achieve their correct weight – and give them slimline eating habits for life. (See also pages 51–58.)

~ Ten good reasons for losing weight with Eat for Life Diet ~

1 It offers permanent weight loss.

The number-one goal of all slimmers is here for the taking. Dieting used to be a vicious circle. In the past dieters returned to the eating habits that caused the weight problem in the first place, and then became stuck in a vicious circle of one diet after another. This is no longer the case. Eat for Life Diet changes your eating habits for ever, allowing you to eat 'normally' for life.

2 Superfoods don't put your health at risk.

Other diets may have relied on one food exclusively, or a limited selection, which leaves the slimmer short of essential nutrients. When cutting down on quantity, it's very important to apply the Eat for Life Diet principle of maintaining top quality by incorporating nutrient-dense superfoods.

3 You will be nicer to live with on this diet.

Other diets have encouraged obsessive behaviour. Dieters can think life is empty or feel they are out of control if they don't stick to difficult diets of deprivation. Eating one chocolate on such a regime creates feelings of guilt that can often lead to giving up in style and eating the whole box – and then abandoning the diet in despair. Self-denial that leads to these feelings is not a feature of Eat for Life Diet because we recognise it only leads to craving, bingeing, and more serious eating problems. On this diet you will not be operating under impossible restrictions, so you won't be irritable, tired and difficult to live with because you won't be hungry and undernourished.

4 You can eat exciting food.

Slimmers can actually eat a wide variety of foods on the Eat for Life Diet. Diets that are unimaginative and boring are doomed to failure for those who love food. However, there are some slimmers who find it easier to eat the same meal three nights a week. Both types are catered for. But if the Easy Option Plan is followed, we suggest that once you have lost weight and got to grips with the simple Eat for Life Diet principles, you return to a more varied pattern of eating.

STRESS-FREE SLIMMING

Because your body will be properly nourished and you will not have to suffer the usual pain and heartache of slimming – hunger pangs, food cravings, irritability, unrealistic demands and expectations of yourself – your stress levels on the Eat for Life Diet will be minimal. The built-in exercise factor will also help keep stress low. Exercise not only speeds up the effect of dieting, it also helps release endorphins (natural brain chemicals) which give a sense of well-being and reduce stress.

CHEESE BORED

Cheese can be the slimmer's downfall because it is high in calories and fat. The answer is to use high-fat cheeses less frequently – perhaps have a cheeseboard only when entertaining. Don't nibble on cheese; it is a meal in itself. For cooking, use well-flavoured, mature cheeses so that a little goes a long way. Especially tasty ones are Farmhouse Cheddar, Gruyère, Emmenthal, Parmesan, Pont l'Eveque, chèvre. Become familiar with lower-fat cheeses such as fromage frais, low-fat curd cheeses and ricotta, and use them in cooking.

HIP, HIP HOORAY

We are not obsessed with hips and thighs. We are not on a mission impossible to change the basic body shape of the female, which has been celebrated from Botticelli to Picasso. Nothing in the world is going to change a pear shape to an hourglass. At any rate, diet won't change your fundamental shape, because that is determined by your genes. Exercise, however, can tone muscles and make you more shapely. Only huff-and-puff can reach the parts that diet can't.

WARNING MUMS TO BE

Unless your doctor has advised you to lose weight, dieting during pregnancy is out of the question. Mothers and babies need calories. You don't need to eat for two – you need only 200 calories a day extra during the last trimester (after 28 weeks) of pregnancy, although if you are underweight at the start of your pregnancy you many need to eat more. Breastfeeding mums need an extra 450-550 calories a day, depending on the age and appetite of the baby. Mums need to eat enough calories to provide the developing baby with protein, iron, calcium, folic acid, vitamin C and some B vitamins, and all those other goodies that are in the Eat for Life Diet. Enjoy the wide variety of foods that provide the nutrients for building muscle, bones, blood, teeth… and all the other ingredients that go into making healthy babies.

5 We never say never again.

Instead of the boring old message of don't eat this and don't eat that, Eat for Life Diet offers a rich array of foods to eat – and lots of them.

6 You can say goodbye to fat hips, stomach and thighs.

Eat for Life Diet makes use of the latest scientific research which shows that calories from fat are more easily converted than calories from CC foods into the fat that causes big hips, thighs and stomach. While meals high in fat encourage body fat to be deposited, meals rich in CC foods encourage calories to be burned off. And if you follow the exercise advice on pages 89–92, the results will be even better.

7 There are no nasty side-effects.

Diets that are very low in calories, such as liquid meal replacements of 600 calories a day or less, might contain the levels of vitamins and minerals that are considered essential for health, but this doesn't mean they are a suitable way to diet. Very low calorie diets and fasting (eating nothing, or just drinking water or fruit juices) result in the body having to burn its own muscle for energy, which is not healthy. These diets also fail to re-educate eating habits. They are a last ditch attempt, and were originally designed for use in hospitals. Very low calorie and crash diets should never be used by teenagers, pregnant or breastfeeding women, or children. And who needs them now that Eat for Life Diet is here?

8 Calories are burned off faster than on many other diets.

Eating more CC foods and fruit and vegetables in place of fatty foods is the most successful way to lose weight. Researchers have proved that the rate at which you burn calories is slowed down by slimming diets that are low in CC foods. This means slimmers put weight back on more easily after a diet that is low in CC foods, because the body needs fewer calories than before. Eat for Life Diet has no such effect: the weight is lost a bit more slowly, but it stays off.

9 Hang on to your muscle power.

When diets go below 1,000 calories they can lead to loss of lean tissue (muscle) rather than fat. This makes it harder to maintain a lower weight because muscle burns calories, and fat doesn't. Exercise builds more calorie-burning muscle; fat just hangs there, looking horrible and irritating you. That's why Eat for Life Diet is based on 1,200 calories a day and incorporates exercise.

10 Our CC fibre doesn't deplete minerals.

The fibre in CC foods 'prolongs gastric emptying' for some people, which is scientific jargon for saying that CC foods make you feel fuller for longer. Because CC foods are bulkier and generally contain fewer calories, slimmers benefit, especially as for some people fibre in starchy foods also decreases the urge to eat. Having the fibre built in to CC foods also prevents problems that may be caused by slimming diets that use a lot of bran. Bran contains substances known as phytates which reduce absorption of minerals such as calcium, iron and zinc.

~ Why lose weight? ~

Having come this far, you probably don't need telling. But the thought of how good you can look when you are the right weight can easily overshadow the health benefits, so it's worth mentioning them once more. Obesity shortens life. It aggravates high blood pressure, heart disease, non-insulin-dependent diabetes, gallstones, gout, osteoarthritis, hiatus hernia, high blood cholesterol. Losing weight reduces raised blood pressure, improves carbohydrate tolerance (good news for non-insulin-dependent diabetics), diminishes osteoarthritis of weight-bearing joints – and helps restore life expectancy to normal.

WEIGHTY REASONS FOR LOW-FAT SLIMMING

The more fat you eat, the more likely you are to have a weight problem. So far, no difference has emerged between saturated and unsaturated fats, as far as weight control is concerned. It is the total amount of fat that needs to be restricted to lose weight. Compare the calories in fat with other foods – and alcohol, which is high in calories.

Calories per gram

Fat:	9 calories per gram
Alcohol:	7 calories per gram
Protein:	4 calories per gram
Carbohydrate:	4 calories per gram

~ The 28-day Slimming Plan ~

1,200 calories per day

The Eat for Life Diet slimming plans fulfill the goals of 50 per cent calories from CC foods; not more than 30 per cent calories from fat. And they're low in saturated fat, sugar and salt.

Daily allowance

300 ml ($^1/_2$ pint) skimmed milk for tea and coffee

or 150 ml ($^1/_4$ pint) skimmed milk and 125 ml (4 fl oz) low-fat natural yogurt

or 200 ml (7 fl oz) soya milk

15 g ($^1/_2$ oz) low-fat spread

or 7 g ($^1/_4$ oz) polyunsaturated margarine

or 15 ml (1 tbsp) French dressing (vinaigrette)

A portion of fresh fruit.

Bread, Rice and Pasta

Bread   Instead of 2 large thick slices of wholemeal bread 100 g ($3^1/_2$ oz); you can use 2 large thick slices of brown, Granary or white bread or 1 large pitta bread or 75 g Ciabatta or 1 large bap.

Rice   50 g (2 oz) uncooked rice = 100 g ($3^1/_2$ oz) cooked rice

Pasta   50 g (2 oz) uncooked pasta = 100 g ($3^1/_2$ oz) cooked pasta

~ Dieting tips ~

- Vegetables should not be tossed in butter, margarine or low-fat spread before serving.
- Keep the use of oil or fat in cooking to a minimum, especially for stir-fried vegetables or browning of meat.
- All spices must be fried before adding any liquid to help develop their flavour, with the exception of those used in marinades.
- Eat larger portions of vegetables if you get hungry.

Note: If you find dieting difficult because you need to snack throughout the day, it is better to eat some fresh fruit or salad as a snack, and then eat the potato, rice, remaining salad and protein part of the meal at the proper time.

PORTIONS OF FRUIT

1 apple
1 small banana
1 orange
1 pear
10 strawberries
1 peach
3 apricots
large slice melon
125 g (4 oz) rasberries
3 plums
10 grapes

BREAKFASTS

WEEK 1

Monday

1 glass fresh orange juice
1 large, thick slice wholemeal toast
scraping of low-fat spread
10 ml (2 tsp) marmalade or jam or
lemon curd

Tuesday

$^1/_2$ grapefruit
45 ml (3 tbsp) bran flakes and milk
from allowance

Wednesday

Apple sliced and mixed with
45 ml (3 tbsp) unsweetened muesli
milk from allowance

Thursday

1 glass fresh orange juice
1 wholemeal muffin
scraping of low-fat spread
yeast extract

Friday

Banana, sliced and mixed with
45 ml (3 tbsp) bran flakes
milk from allowance

Saturday

1 glass fresh orange juice
1 large, thick slice Granary bread
1 small slice lean ham
or 1 small cheese triangle

Sunday

$^1/_2$ grapefruit
1 large, thick slice wholemeal toast
mushrooms cooked 10 g ($^1/_3$ oz) low-fat
spread in non-stick pan.

WEEK 2

Monday

2 wholewheat biscuits with 15 ml (1 tbsp)
raisins
milk from allowance

Tuesday

1 glass fresh orange juice
1 large, thick slice wholemeal toast
1 triangle cheese spread

Wednesday

$^1/_2$ grapefruit
40 g ($1^1/_2$ oz) porridge oats made with water
milk from allowance
10 ml (2 tsp) brown sugar or honey

Thursday

1 glass fresh orange juice
1 wholemeal hot-cross bun – warmed in the
microwave or toasted
scraping of low-fat spread

Friday

1 banana
1 large thick slice wholemeal toast
10 ml (2 tsp) citrus spread

Saturday

1 glass fresh orange juice
45 ml (3 tbsp) muesli mixed with
a chopped apple
milk from allowance

Sunday

$^1/_2$ grapefruit
1 large, thick slice wholemeal toast
1 poached or boiled egg
scraping of low-fat spread

WEEK 3

Monday

1 glass fresh orange juice
45 ml (3 tbsp) unsweetened muesli
milk from allowance

Tuesday

$^{1}/_{2}$ grapefruit
1 large, thick slice wholemeal toast
scraping of low-fat spread
yeast extract

Wednesday

45 ml (3 tbsp) bran flakes
1 banana, sliced
milk from allowance

Thursday

1 glass fresh orange juice
1 wholemeal hot cross bun
scraping of low-fat spread

Friday

1 apple
1 wholemeal muffin
scraping of low-fat spread
10 ml (2 tsp) marmalade or jam
or lemon curd

Saturday

1 glass orange juice
1 slice wholemeal toast
2 halves grilled tomatoes
50 g (2 oz) mushrooms cooked in a
scraping of low-fat spread

Sunday

$^{1}/_{2}$ grapefruit
1 slice wholemeal toast
1 rasher grilled back bacon
Vegetarian option: 1 poached egg

WEEK 4

Monday

1 glass fresh orange juice
40 g ($1^{1}/_{2}$ oz) porridge oats made with water
milk from allowance
10 ml (2 tsp) brown sugar or honey

Tuesday

1 banana
1 large, thick slice wholemeal toast
scraping of low-fat spread
10 ml (2 tsp) marmalade or jam
or lemon curd

Wednesday

45 ml (3 tbsp) muesli mixed with
1 chopped apple
milk from allowance

Thursday

1 glass fresh orange juice
1 wholemeal muffin
scaping of low-fat spread
10 ml (2 tsp) marmalade or jam
or lemon curd

Friday

1 apple
2 wholewheat biscuits
milk from allowance

Saturday

1 glass fresh orange juice
1 poached egg on one large slice wholemeal
toast scraping of low-fat spread

Sunday

1 glass fresh orange juice
sliced tomato and cheese on toast

LUNCHES

*★ Recipes for dishes marked with a star may be found
in the recipe chapter. See pages 101–146.*

WEEK 1

Monday

50 g (2 oz) lean roast chicken meat and
Italian Salad★ sandwich made with 2 large,
thick slices wholemeal bread
1 apple
Vegetarian option: 1 hard-boiled egg,
sliced, and Italian Salad★ sandwich made
with 2 large, thick slices wholemeal bread
1 apple

Tuesday

175 g (6 oz) jacket potato filled with 150 g
(5 oz) baked beans and 25 g (1 oz) lean ham
and chopped tomato salad
1 banana
Vegetarian option: 175 g (6 oz) jacket
potato filled with 150 g (5 oz) baked beans
and 15 g (1/2 oz) Parmesan cheese and
chopped tomato salad
1 banana

Wednesday

Mexican Tuna★ salad sandwich made with
2 large, thick slices Granary bread and
an extra tomato
1 orange
Vegetarian option: 50 g (2 oz) Hummus★
salad sandwich made with 2 large, thick
slices of Granary bread
1 orange

Thursday

50 g (2 oz) reduced-fat hard cheese and
salad sandwich made with a
large brown bap
1 pear

Friday

175 g (6 oz) jacket potato with 75 g (3 oz)
cottage cheese, grated carrots
and 15 g (1/2 oz) nuts
1 portion fresh fruit salad

Saturday

Bean Soup★
1 wholemeal roll
1 apple

Sunday

100 g (3 1/2 oz) lean roast leg of lamb
Ratatouille★ peas
100 g (3 1/2 oz) cooked basmati rice
Fruit Kebabs★
Vegetarian option: 50 g (2 oz) reduced-
fat hard cheese with 100 g (3 1/2 oz) cooked
basmati rice, Ratatouille★, peas
Fruit Kebabs★

WEEK 2

Monday

150 g (5 oz) vegetarian pizza
tomato and pepper salad
1 pear

Tuesday

50 g (2 oz) lean ham, and Winter Salad★
sandwich made with 2 large, thick slices
wholemeal bread
1 apple
Vegetarian option: 50 g (2 oz) Hummus★
and Winter Salad★ sandwich made with
2 large, thick slices wholemeal bread
1 apple

Wednesday

50 g (2 oz) sardine and tomato sandwich
made with 2 large, thick slices
wholemeal bread
1 orange
Vegetarian option: cucumber raita
and Bean Salad★ and pitta bread
1 orange

Thursday

175 g (6 oz) jacket potato filled
with 50 g (2 oz) reduced-fat hard cheese
and grated carrot
1 apple

Friday

Pan Bagnet : Egg, Tuna and Black Olive
Salad★ sandwich made with a large piece
of French bread
1 banana
Vegetarian option: Egg and Black Olive
Salad★ sandwich made with a large piece
of French bread
1 banana

Saturday

Avocado, Prawn and Celery Salad★
1 wholemeal roll
cherries
Vegetarian option: Avocado,
Walnut and Celery Salad★
1 wholemeal roll
cherries

Sunday

75 g (3 oz) roast chicken, no skin
175 g (6 oz) boiled potato
broccoli
carrots
Fresh Fruit Platter with Mango Sauce★
Vegetarian option: 1 portion
Lazy Lentils★
150 g (5 oz) boiled potatoes
broccoli
carrots
Fresh Fruit Platter with Mango Sauce★

WEEK 3

Monday

Toasted sandwich made with 50 g (2 oz)
reduced-fat grated cheese and 2 large, thick
slices wholemeal bread and salad
1 banana

Tuesday

3 oz (75 g) chicken and Turkish Salad★
sandwich, made with 2 large, thick slices of
Granary bread
1 pear
Vegetarian option: peanut butter and
Turkish Salad★ sandwich made with 2 large,
thick slices of Granary bread
1 pear

Wednesday

50 g (2 oz) Aubergine Pâté ★
with wholemeal pitta bread
tomato and cucumber salad
1 apple

Thursday

Egg and Watercress Salad★
sandwich made with 2 large, thick
slices wholemeal bread
1 peach

Friday

50 g (2 oz) Smoked Mackerel Pâté★
with 2 large, thick slices
wholemeal toast
Fennel, Apricot and Walnut Salad★
1 apple
Vegetarian option: 50 g (2 oz) Bean
Pâté★
with 2 large, thick
slices wholemeal toast
Fennel, Apricot and Walnut Salad★
1 apple

─────── *Saturday* ───────

Chicken and blue cheese American
Sandwich★ and salad
grapes
Vegetarian option: American Sandwich★
made with 40 g (1¹/₂ oz)
blue cheese instead of chicken
grapes

─────── *Sunday* ───────

75 g (3 oz) lean roast pork
red cabbage
175 g (6 oz) boiled new potatoes
green beans
small portion Cheesecake★
with Rhubarb Sauce★
Vegetarian option: Leek Risotto★
green beans
small portion Cheesecake★
and Rhubarb Sauce★

WEEK 4

─────── *Monday* ───────

Crab and Lemon Coleslaw★ sandwich made
with 2 large, thick slices wholemeal bread
1 apple
Vegetarian option: 50 g (2 oz)
Hummus★ with Lemon Coleslaw★
sandwich made with 2 large, thick slices
wholemeal bread
1 apple

─────── *Tuesday* ───────

50 g (2 oz) lean roast beef with Italian
Salad★ and 5 ml (1 tsp) horseradish
sandwich made with
2 large, thick slices wholemeal bread
1 nectarine
Vegetarian option: Bean Soup★ with 2
large thick slices wholemeal toast and
Italian Salad★
1 nectarine

─────── *Wednesday* ───────

50 g (2 oz) prawns with Winter Salad★ in 1
wholemeal pitta bread
1 orange
Vegetarian option: 150 g (5 oz)
vegetarian wholemeal pizza and
Winter Salad★
1 orange

─────── *Thursday* ───────

Tabbouleh★ and chicken sandwich made
with 2 large, thick slices wholemeal bread
1 banana
Vegetarian option: Tabbouleh★ sandwich
made with 25 g (1 oz) chopped nuts instead
of chicken, and 2 large,
thick slices wholemeal bread
1 banana

─────── *Friday* ───────

Wholemeal Pasta Salad★ with green salad
3 plums
Vegetarian option: Vegetarian
Wholemeal Pasta Salad★ made with 50 g
(2 oz) reduced-fat cheese per person instead
of crab, with green salad
3 plums

─────── *Saturday* ───────

Vegetables, Bean and Pasta Soup★ and a
wholemeal roll, served with 15 g (¹/₂ oz)
Parmesan cheese
¹/₂ sliced orange and ¹/₂ sliced banana

─────── *Sunday* ───────

100 g (3¹/₂ oz) Roast beef
175 g (6 oz) boiled potatoes
cabbage
carrots
Walnut Stuffed Pears★ with
15 ml (1 tbsp) Greek yoghurt
Vegetarian option: Chick Pea Hot Pot★
175 g (6 oz) boiled potatoes
cabbage
carrots
Walnut Stuffed Pears★ with
15 ml (1 tbsp) Greek yoghurt

EVENING MEALS

WEEK 1

Monday

Butterbean and Mushroom Bake★
175 g (6 oz) jacket potato
grated carrot salad
tomato salad
1 glass fresh orange juice

Tuesday

Chicken in Watercress Sauce★
100 g (3½ oz) cooked pasta
broccoli
carrots
Pear with Fresh Ginger★
Vegetarian option: 1 Stuffed Pepper★
broccoli
carrots
a bread roll
Pear with Fresh Ginger★

Wednesday

100 g (3½ oz) cooked spicy rice
100 g (3½ oz) fish or chicken tikka kebab
made with 100 g (3½ oz)
Fish and Tikka Marinade★
Turkish Salad★
lettuce
1 fresh mango
Vegetarian option: 225 g (8 oz)
Vegetarian Chilli★
100 g (3½ oz) cooked spicy rice
Turkish Salad★
lettuce
1 fresh mango

Thursday

Pasta with Aubergine and Tomato Sauce★
mixed salad
1 scoop Lemon Sorbet★

Friday

100 g (3½ oz) boiled rice
Stir-fried Vegetables★ made with
75 g (3 oz) pork
baked apple with raisins and
low-fat yogurt from allowance
Vegetarian option: Stir-fried Vegetables★
with
25 g (1 oz) flaked toasted almonds
100 g (3½ oz) boiled rice
baked apple and raisins and
low-fat yogurt from allowance

Saturday

175 g (6 oz) boiled new potatoes
green beans and Tomato Sauce★
100 g (3½ oz) baked salmon
Peach Brûlée★
Vegetarian option: Spinach Squares★
175 g (6 oz) boiled new potatoes
green beans and Tomato Sauce★
Peach Brûlée★

Sunday

50 g (2 oz) Bean Pâté★ and pitta bread
with green salad
grapes

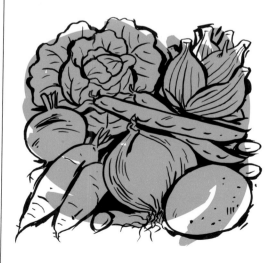

WEEK 2

Monday

Fish and Vegetable Kebab★
175 g (6 oz) boiled potatoes
broccoli
raspberries and $\frac{1}{2}$ banana
Vegetarian option: Vegetable Tortilla★,
75 g (3 oz) boiled potatoes
broccoli
carrots
raspberries and $\frac{1}{2}$ banana

Tuesday

Keema★
100 g ($3\frac{1}{2}$ oz) cooked boiled rice
carrot salad
tomato salad
1 apple
Vegetarian option: Spinach and Lentil
Dhansak★
100 g ($3\frac{1}{2}$ oz) cooked boiled rice
carrot salad
tomato salad
1 apple

Wednesday

Pasta with Liver★
fennel and tomato salad
1 slice fresh pineapple
Vegetarian option: 100 g ($3\frac{1}{2}$ oz) cooked
pasta with spicy tomato sauce
(Tomato Sauce★ heated with 1 dried chilli)
fennel and tomato salad
1 slice fresh pineapple

Thursday

75 g (3 oz) lean roast chicken
Indian Potatoes★
carrots
peas
Fresh Fruit Platter★
Vegetarian option: Chick Pea Hot Pot★
Indian Potatoes★
carrots
peas
Fresh Fruit Platter★

Friday

grilled 175 g (6 oz) trout
175 g (6 oz) boiled potatoes
peas
baked tomatoes with herbs
Fresh Fruit Baked in Foil Parcels★
Vegetarian option: Courgette Goulash★
175 g (6 oz) boiled potatoes
peas
tomatoes
Fresh Fruit Baked in Foil Parcels★

Saturday

grilled 100 g ($3\frac{1}{2}$ oz) pork chop, trimmed
of fat, with Red Pepper Sauce★
175 g (6 oz) boiled potatoes
Poppyseed Leeks★
carrots
1 scoop Strawberry Yogurt Ice Cream★
Vegetarian option: Pasta with
Beans and Mushrooms★
Poppyseed Leeks★
carrots
1 scoop Strawberry Yogurt Ice Cream★

Sunday

Pasta ai Funghi★
green salad
Dried Fruit Salad★

WEEK 3

Monday

Nasi Goreng★
tomato and cucumber salad
sprouted lentil salad or green salad
3 plums
Vegetarian option: Nasi Goreng★ without
the meat but served with an omelette
(using 1 egg per person)
tomato and cucumber salad
sprouted lentil salad
3 plums

Tuesday

grilled tuna steak
Tomato Salsa★
carrot salad
¼ of a large baguette
Fruit Kebabs★
Vegetarian option: Hungarian Potatoes★
carrot salad
¼ of a large baguette
Fruit Kebabs★

Wednesday

grilled chicken
(marinaded in Soy Sauce Marinade★ if
desired)
100 g (3½ oz) Lemon Rice★
green beans and Tomato Sauce★
sweetcorn
blackberries and apple
Vegetarian option: green beans and
Tomato Sauce★
100 g (3½ oz) Lemon Rice★ with
25 g (1 oz) chopped cashews
sweetcorn
Raita★
blackberries and apple

Thursday

Kedgeree★
tomato salad
Bean Salad★
kiwi fruit
Vegetarian option: Leek Risotto★
Bean Salad★
tomato salad
kiwi fruit

Friday

Pork and Bean Goulash★
175 g (6 oz) jacket potato
green beans
1 scoop Rhubarb Sorbet★
Vegetarian option: Bean Goulash★
175 g (6 oz) jacket potato
green beans
1 scoop Rhubarb Sorbet★

Saturday

Spicy Lamb with Chickpeas and Apricots★
(replace chicken with lamb in chickpea,
chicken and apricot dish)
100 g (3½ oz) Persian Rice★
Turkish Salad★
green salad
Pears with Fresh Ginger★
Vegetarian option: Spicy Chickpeas and
Apricots★
100 g (3½ oz) Persian Rice★
Turkish Salad★
green salad
Pears with Fresh Ginger★

Sunday

Salad Niçoise ★
Granary bread
1 apple
Vegetarian option: Vegetarian Salad
Niáoise★ (made without the tuna)
Granary bread
1 apple

WEEK 4

Monday

Fish Soup★
1 bread roll
mixed salad
1 slice fresh pineapple
Vegetarian option: Lentil and Spinach
Soup★
1 bread roll
mixed salad
1 slice fresh pineapple

Tuesday

Grilled home-made hamburger,
with Tomato Sauce★ (optional)
100 g (3¹/₂ oz) Spicy Rice★
green salad
carrot salad
baked banana with yogurt from allowance
Vegetarian option: Mange Tout Stir Fry★
100 g (3¹/₂ oz) Spicy Rice★
green salad
carrot salad
baked banana with yogurt from allowance

Wednesday

Seafood Salad★
bread roll
cucumber salad
tomato salad
melon and strawberries
Vegetarian option: Spinach Squares★
1 bread roll
cucumber salad
tomato salad
melon and strawberries

Thursday

100 g (3¹/₂ oz) roast pork
175 g (6 oz) boiled potatoes
Italian Cabbage★
peas
peaches and rasberries
Vegetarian option: Butterbean and
Mushroom Bake★
175 g (6 oz) boiled potatoes
Italian Cabbage★
peas
peaches and raspberries

Friday

Spicy Chicken Noodles★
Garden Salad★
Mango Salsa★
fresh fruit salad
Vegetarian option: Spicy Noodles★
made with 25 g (1 oz) chopped peanuts
instead of the chicken
Garden Salad★
Mango Salsa★
fresh fruit salad

Saturday

Seafood Risotto★
Watercress and Orange Salad★
Mushroom Salad★
Peach Stuffed with Almonds★
Vegetarian option: Courgette Risotto★
Watercress and Orange Salad★
Mushroom Salad★
Peaches Stuffed with Almonds★

Sunday

150 g (5 oz) vegetarian pizza
Carrot and Nut Salad★
tomato salad
1 slice of pineapple

~ Easy Option Slimming Plan ~

There never seems to be enough time in the day to do everything that needs to be done – let alone think about losing weight! The Easy Option Plan is designed with you in mind. All you need to do is choose one of the breakfasts, one of the lunches and an evening meal. If you prefer to eat breakfast at mid-morning instead of first thing, it is entirely up to you. Although you could eat pasta and tomato sauce every night, we wouldn't recommend it! Any diet is much healthier and more nutritious if you vary it as much as possible.

Although we haven't stated portion sizes we would suggest the following:

1   Use large thick slices of bread for sandwiches and breakfast.
2   Choose reduced-fat hard cheeses instead of high-fat cheeses.
3   Use the minimum amount of filling, except for salad, for the sandwiches – 50 g (2 oz) of meat, fish, pâté, cheese or egg.
4   We need the following portion sizes for the CC foods: 50 g (2 oz) uncooked pasta or 100 g (3^1/2 oz) cooked pasta; 50 g (2 oz) uncooked rice or 100 g (3^1/2 oz) cooked rice or 175 g (6 oz) cooked potato or 2 large, thick slices of bread. Try to use wholemeal varieties as much as possible, but that doesn't mean you can't use white rice, pasta or bread.
5   Always choose lean meat and keep the portion size small.

Daily allowance

300 ml (^{1}/2 pint) skimmed milk

  or 150 ml (^{1}/4 pint) skimmed milk and 150 ml (5 fl oz) low-fat yogurt.

15 g (^{1}/2 oz) low-fat spread

  or 5 ml (1 tsp) oil

  or 7.5 ml (^{1}/2 tbsp) French dressing;

  or 7 g (^{1}/4 oz) polyunsaturated margarine.

A portion of fresh fruit.

BREAKFAST

1 slice wholemeal toast and scraping low-fat spread from allowance and 1 small slice lean ham and 1 portion fruit

1 slice granary toast and 1 triangle cheese spread and 1 portion fruit

45 ml (3 tbsp) bran flakes and milk fron allowance and 1 portion fruit

2 Weetabix and milk from allowance and 1 portion fruit

2 Shredded Wheat and milk from allowance and 1 portion of fruit

1 slice wholemeal toast and 10 ml (2 tsp) peanut butter and 1 portion fruit

45 ml (3 tbsp) muesli and milk from allowance and 1 portion fruit

1 wholemeal hot-cross bun and scraping low-fat spread from allowance and 1 portion fruit

1 slice brown bread and scraping low-fat spread from allowance and 1 portion fruit

1 slice wholemeal bread and scraping low-fat spread from allowance and 10 ml (2 tsp) jam or marmalade or lemon curd and 1 portion of fruit

1 slice rye bread and 2 halves grilled tomato and 50 g (2 oz) mushrooms cooked in 2.5 ml (^{1}/2 tsp) low-fat spread from allowance and 1 portion fruit

40 g (1^1/2 oz) porridge oats made with water, 10 ml (2 tsp) brown sugar, milk from allowance and 1 portion fruit

1 slice wholemeal bread, scraping low-fat spread from allowance and 1 poached egg and 1 portion fruit

1 wholemeal muffin and scraping low-fat spread from allowance and 10 ml (2 tsp) jam or marmalade or lemon curd and 1 portion fruit

LUNCH

Small slice vegetarian pizza and 1 portion fruit

Cheese and salad sandwich and 1 portion fruit

Roast beef and horseradish and salad sandwich and 1 portion of fruit

Roast chicken and Italian Salad★ sandwich and 1 portion of fruit

Hummus and salad and pitta bread and 1 portion fruit

Egg and Watercress Sandwich★ and 1 portion fruit

Pasta, Bean and Vegetable Soup★ and 1 wholemeal roll and 1 portion fruit

Tomato and Courgette Soup★ and 1 bread roll and reduced-fat cheese and 1 portion fruit

Ham and salad sandwich and 1 portion fruit

Sardine, tomato and lettuce sandwich and 1 portion fruit

Egg and Black Olive Salad★ sandwich and 1 portion fruit
Peanut butter and salad sandwich and 1 portion fruit

Smoked Mackerel Pâté★ and salad and pitta bread and 1 portion fruit

Aubergine Pâté★ and pitta bread, salad
and 1 portion fruit

40 g (1¹/2 oz) blue cheese and tomato
toasted sandwich, salad and 1 portion fruit

Curried chicken toasted sandwich, made
with 50 g (2 oz) lean roast chicken,
10 g (¹/3 oz) reduced-fat mayonnaise, 10 g
(¹/3 oz) low-fat yogurt, 2.5 ml (¹/2 tsp) jam
and a pinch of curry powder; salad and
1 portion fruit

Prawns and Winter Salad★ and 75 g (3 oz)
Ciabatta and 1 portion fruit

Pork and Cabbage Salad★ sandwich
and 1 portion fruit

Mexican Tuna★ and salad sandwich
and 1 portion fruit

Summer Soup and 1 bread roll, cheese salad
and 1 portion fruit

Jacket potato with cottage cheese and grated
carrots and 25 g (1 oz) nuts and
1 portion fruit

Jacket potato with baked beans and salad
and 1 portion fruit

Jacket potato with small portion chilli con
carne and salad and 1 portion fruit

Jacket potato with cheese and salad
and 1 portion fruit

Jacket potato with Provençale sauce
(Tomato Sauce★ and 50 g (2 oz) prawns
cooked together) and salad and
1 portion fruit

Jacket potato with Ratatouille★
and 1 portion fruit

Cheese and Turkish Salad★ sandwich
and 1 portion fruit

Chicken and Tabbouleh★ sandwich
and 1 portion fruit

Salad Niçoise★ and 1 bread roll
and 1 portion fruit

Thai Chicken★ salad and 1 bread roll
and 1 portion fruit

Broad bean, cheese, pepper and lettuce salad
and 1 bread roll and 1 portion fruit

Spinach and Ham Salad★ and 1 granary roll
and 1 portion fruit

Brown Rice Salad★ and 1 portion fruit

Tuna Bean Salad★ and 1 bread roll
and 1 portion fruit

EVENING

Rice with Keema★ and 2 salads
and 1 portion fruit

Pasta with bolognaise sauce and 2 salads
and 1 portion fruit

Rice and stir-fried liver and 2 vegetables
and 1 portion fruit

Rice with chicken tikka and 2 salads
and 1 portion fruit

Pasta and Aubergine Sauce★ and mozzarella
cheese and 1 salad and 1 portion fruit

Boiled potato and 100 g (3¹/2 oz) grilled
pork chop with the fat removed and
2 vegetables and 1 portion fruit

Jacket potato and chicken with large
portion Stir-fried Vegetables★ and
1 portion fruit

Rice with beef and Stir-fried Vegetables★
and one salad and 1 portion fruit

Pasta with Provençale sauce (Tomato
Sauce★ and prawns and cod) and one salad
and 1 portion fruit

Rice with Ratatouille★ and cheese and one
salad and 1 portion fruit

Pasta with small portion Tomato Sauce★
cooked with mushrooms and pork chop and
one salad and 1 portion fruit

Boiled potato with lemon chicken (small
breast of chicken cooked in Lemon
Marinade★) and 2 vegetables
and 1 portion fruit

Pasta with Red Pepper Sauce★ and 15 g
(^{1}/2 oz) Parmesan cheese and salad
and 1 portion fruit

Spicy Rice★ with 75 g (3 oz) lean leg of
lamb and vegetable kebab and one vegetable
and 1 portion fruit

Boiled potato with grilled trout and 2
vegetables and 1 portion fruit

Pasta with Kidney Beans and Bacon★
and 2 salads and 1 portion fruit

Tuna Bake★ and 2 vegetables
and 1 portion fruit

Boiled potato, 100 g (3^1/2 oz) grilled rump
steak and 2 salads and 1 portion fruit

Rice with Stir-fried Vegetables★ and
15 g (^{1}/2 oz) flaked almonds and 25 g (1 oz)
reduced-fat hard cheese, grated,
and 1 portion fruit

Pasta with Courgette Goulash★ and one
salad and 1 portion fruit

Boiled potatoes, 125 g (4 oz) baked salmon
and 2 vegetables 1 portion fruit

Rice with Ratatouille★, 75 g (3 oz) lean
roast leg lamb and 1 vegetable
and 1 portion fruit

Chick Pea Hot Pot★ and rice and 2 salads
and 1 portion fruit

Rice, 125 g (4 oz) grilled hamburger and
2 salads and 1 portion fruit

Jacket potato, Lazy Lentils★ and 2 salads
and 1 portion fruit

Hungarian Potatoes★, 100 g (3^1/2 oz)
grilled pork chop with the fat removed and
2 vegetables and 1 portion fruit

Pasta with Beans and Prawns★ and one salad
and 1 portion fruit

Leek Risotto★ and 2 salads
and 1 portion fruit

Pasta ai Funghi★ and 2 salads
and 1 portion fruit

Rice with small chicken breast cooked in
Red Pepper Sauce★ and one salad
and 1 portion fruit

Boiled potato, Spicy Fish Tikka★ and 2
salads and 1 portion fruit

Jacket potato, 100 g (3^1/2 oz) grilled leg of
lamb with the fat removed and 2 vegetables
and 1 portion of fruit

Boiled potato, 75 g (3 oz) roast chicken, no
skin, and 2 vegetables and 1 portion fruit

USING MANUFACTURED FOODS

Sometimes, preparing food can seem like too much effort, particularly when you are trying to diet. To help you diet the Easy Option Plan allows you to choose an occasional readymade meal as an alternative to cooking. However, some of these dishes are higher in fat and more expensive than food prepared at home, so we certainly don't suggest that you use them all the time.

LUNCH

Try to choose a sandwich that has plenty of salad, and always have a piece of fruit. Here are sandwiches made by various manufacturers that you can eat on your diet. They all contain less than 300 calories.

Boots Shapers:

Smoked ham, soft cheese and pineapple with lettuce – 222 Calories
Turkey and Chinese leaf with sage and onion mayonnaise – 237 Calories
Cheese and celery with mayonnaise – 250 Calories
Chicken and Chinese leaf and lemon mayonnaise – 250 Calories
Tuna, mayonnaise and cucumber – 205 Calories
Prawn, apple and celery with mayonnaise – 264 Calories
Cheese crunch with carrot, celery, almonds and yogurt dressing – 271 Calories
Poached salmon and Chinese leaf with mayonnaise – 261 Calories
Barbeque chicken with smoky barbecue mayonnaise and lettuce – 259 Calories

Sainsbury:

Salmon and cucumber – less than 300 Calories
Roast beef and horseradish – less than 300 Calories
Prawns and reduced-calorie mayonnaise – less than 300 Calories

Tesco:

Healthy Eating beef and salad – 240 Calories
Healthy Eating tuna and cucumber – 264 Calories
Oak-smoked ham with salad – 277 Calories

Marks and Spencer:

Prawn and cucumber dressing – 233 Calories
Egg and cress – 297 Calories
Chicken and grape – 255 Calories

EVENING

Readymade meals have revolutionised many of our lives. No longer is the sole choice between cooking foods at home or eating out. We can now eat readymade meals that require minimal preparation. However, research has shown that if we eat these dishes we may not eat vegetables with them. In line with the Eat for Life Diet principles, you should try to have at least two vegetables or salads in the evening and a piece of fruit with your meal. So choose a readymade meal with no more than 450 Calories – including rice, pasta or potato.

Sainsbury:

Frozen Meals

Quick Cuisine chilli con carne with rice – 195 Calories
Quick Cuisine vegetable pasta provencal – 150 Calories
Quick Cuisine sweet and sour chicken with rice – 270 Calories
Healthy Cuisine zucchini lasagne – 340 Calories
Healthy Cuisine vegetable chilli – 305 Calories
Healthy Cuisine chicken madras - 403 Calories
Healthy Cuisine chicken à l'orange – 326 Calories

Healthy Cuisine glazed chicken – 370 Calories

Spaghetti bolognaise – 285 Calories

Chilled Meals

Mushroom and ricotta cannelloni – 390 Calories per serving

Chicken korma with turmeric rice – 270 Calories

Tagliatelle with fresh vegetables – 320 Calories

Potato, leek and celery bake – 245 Calories per serving

Cumberland cottage pie – 290 Calories per serving

Lasagne – 365 Calories

Vegetable lasagne – 340 Calories

Tesco:

Beef Stew and Dumplings – 300 Calories

Tagliatelle Carbonara – 378 Calories

Frozen Meals

Healthy Eating chicken supreme with rice – 395 Calories

Italian chicken pasta snack – 385 Calories

Healthy Eating ocean pie – 391 Calories

Vegetable lasagne – 335 Calories

Chilled Meals

Leek and potato bake – 170 Calories

Spaghetti bolognaise – 266 Calories

Tuna and pasta salad – 387 Calories

Lancashire hot pot – 200 Calories

Chilli con carne – 255 Calories

Safeway:

Frozen Meals

Shepherds Pie – 253 Calories

Chinese style stir fry – 241 Calories (Add 100g (4 oz) boiled rice)

Roast beef in gravy – 207 Calories (Add 175 g (6 oz) boiled potatoes)

Macaroni cheese with ham – 415 Calories

Chilled Meals

Vegetable stir fry with beef – 224 Calories (Add 100 g (3^1/2 oz) boiled rice)

Vegetable chilli – 143 Calories (Add 100 g (3^1/2 oz) boiled rice)

Lasagne – 444 Calories

Moussaka – 384 Calories

Microwave Meals

Pasta bolognaise – 273 Calories

Beef stew with dumplings – 303 Calories

Moussaka – 336 Calories

Birds Eye:

Healthy Options vegetable bolognaise – 370 Calories

Healthy Options vegetable tandoori curry and rice – 395 Calories

Healthy Options vegetable lasagne – 305 Calories

Findus:

Lean Cuisine glazed chicken with rice – less than 300 Calories

Lean Cuisine sesame chicken and fried rice – less than 300 Calories

Lean Cuisine lamb tikka masala and rice – less than 300 Calories

Lean Cuisine chicken and prawn cantonese – less than 300 Calories

Lean Cuisine spicy chicken creole – less than 300 Calories

Heinz:

Weight Watchers pasta shells with vegetables and prawns – 225 Calories

Weight Watchers vegetable moussaka – 157 Calories

Weight Watchers vegetable curry and rice – 286 Calories

Weight Watchers chicken marengo and rice – 272 Calories

Weight Watchers vegetable canneloni – 212 Calories

Boots:

Shapers pasta bolognaise – 262 Calories

Shapers ham and mushroom lasagne – 281 Calories

Shapers tagliatelle carbonara – 298 Calories

Shapers chicken supreme – 260 Calories

Shapers chicken curry and rice – 254 Calories

T

Everyday 7-Day 2,000 Calorie Eating Plan

his diet has been developed to show how you could adapt the 28–Day Slimming Plan (which is 1,200 Calories per day) once you have stopped dieting, or for another member of your family who is not on a diet. Most of us eat and drink more when we are at home, so the calorie intake is more generous at the weekend and more stringent during the week.

Daily allowance
300 ml (1/2 pint) skimmed or semi–skimmed milk
   or 150 ml (1/4 pint) skimmed milk and 100 ml (4 fl oz) low–fat natural yogurt
   or 200 ml (7 fl oz) soya milk.
15 g (1/2 oz) polyunsaturated margarine
   or 25 g (1 oz) low–fat polyunsaturated oil
   or 15 ml (1 tbsp) French dressing.
A portion of fresh fruit.

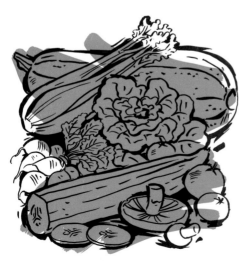

BREAKFAST

Monday

1 glass fresh orange juice
1 large, thick slice wholemeal toast
scraping of polyunsaturated margarine
10 ml (2 tsp) marmalade or jam
or lemon curd
45 ml (3 tbsp) bran flakes

Tuesday

1/2 grapefruit
45 ml (3 tbsp) bran flakes,
milk from allowance
1 large, thick slice Granary bread
scraping of polyunsaturated margarine
10 ml (2 tsp) marmalade or jam
or lemon curd

Wednesday

1 apple sliced and mixed with 45 ml (3 tbsp)
unsweetened museli
milk from allowance
1 large, thick slice wholemeal bread
scraping of polyunsaturated margarine
10 ml (2 tsp) marmalade or jam
or lemon curd

Thursday

1 glass fresh orange juice
1 wholemeal muffin
scraping of polyunsaturated margarine
yeast extract
2 Weetabix
milk from allowance

Friday

1 banana, sliced and mixed with
45 ml (3 tbsp) bran flakes
milk from allowance
1 large thick slice wholemeal bread
scraping of polyunsaturated margarine
10 ml (2 tsp) marmalade or jam
or lemon curd

Saturday

1 glass fresh orange juice
1 large, thick slice Granary bread
1 small slice lean ham or
1 small cheese triangle
45 ml (3 tbsp) bran flakes
milk from allowance

Sunday

1/2 grapefruit
2 large, thick slices wholemeal toast
mushrooms cooked with 7 g (1/4 oz)
polyunsaturated spread in non-stick pan
2 small rashers lean back bacon, grilled
Vegetarian option: 1 poached egg

LUNCHES

Monday

50 g (2 oz) lean roast chicken meat and
Italian Salad★ sandwich made with 2 large,
thick slices wholemeal bread
1 apple
Vegetarian option: 1 hard-boiled egg,
sliced and Italian Salad★ sandwich made
with 2 large, thick slices wholemeal bread
1 apple

Tuesday

225 g (8 oz) jacket potato filled with 150 g
(5 oz) baked beans and 50 g (2 oz) lean ham
and chopped tomato salad
1 banana
Vegetarian option: 225 g (8 oz) jacket
potato filled with 150 g (5 oz) baked beans
and 15 g (1/2 oz) Parmesan cheese and
chopped tomato salad
1 banana

Wednesday

Mexican Tuna★ salad sandwich made with
2 large, thick slices Granary bread
and an extra tomato
1 orange
Vegetarian option: 50 g (2 oz) Hummus★
salad sandwich made with 2 large,
thick slices Granary bread
1 orange

Thursday

50 g (2 oz) reduced-fat hard cheese and
salad sandwich made from a
large brown bap
1 pear
1 low-fat fruit yogurt

Friday

175 g (6 oz) jacket potato with 75 g (3 oz)
cottage cheese, grated carrots and
15 g (1/2 oz) nuts
1 portion fresh fruit salad

Saturday

Bean Soup★
ham and salad sandwich made with
2 large, thick slices wholemeal bread
and 50 g (2 oz) lean ham
1 apple
Vegetarian option: Bean Soup★
pitta bread filled with salad and
50 g (2 oz) grated Edam cheese
1 apple

Sunday

100 g (3 1/2 oz) lean roast leg of lamb
Ratatouille★
peas
200 g (7 oz) cooked basmati rice
Fruit Kebabs★
Vegetarian option: 50 g (2 oz) reduced-
fat hard cheese
200 g (7 oz) cooked basmati rice
Ratatouille★
peas
Fruit Kebabs★

MID-AFTERNOON SNACKS

Tuesday

2 digestive biscuits

Thursday

1 sultana scone with scraping of butter

Saturday

1 large slice chocolate cake with
buttercream icing

EVENING

Monday

Butterbean and Mushroom★ bake
grated carrot salad
tomato salad
225 g (8 oz) jacket potato
1 glass fresh orange juice
1 low-fat fruit yogurt

Tuesday

Chicken in Watercress Sauce★
200 g (7 oz) cooked pasta
broccoli
carrots
Pear with Fresh Ginger★
2 glasses dry white wine
Vegetarian option: 1 large Stuffed
Pepper★
broccoli
carrots
1 bread roll
Pear with Fresh Ginger★
2 glasses dry white wine

Wednesday

100 g (3½ oz) fish or chicken tikka kebab
made with 100 g
(3½ oz) Fish and Tikka Marinade★
150 g (5 oz) oven chips
Turkish Salad★
lettuce
fresh mango and 1 scoop raspberry sorbet
Vegetarian option: 225 g (8 oz)
Vegetarian Chilli★
200 g (7 oz) cooked spicy rice
Turkish Salad★
lettuce
fresh mango and 1 scoop raspberry sorbet

Thursday

Pasta with Aubergine and Tomato Sauce★
mixed salad
winter salad
2 scoops lemon Sorbet★
2 glasses red wine

Friday

200 g (7 oz) boiled rice
Stir-fried Vegetables★ with 75 g (3 oz) pork
baked apple with raisins and
low-fat yogurt from allowance
1 small glass of lager
Vegetarian option: Stir-fried Vegetables★
with 25 g (1 oz)
flaked toasted almonds
200 g (7 oz) boiled rice
baked apple and raisins and
low-fat yogurt from allowance
1 small glass of lager

Saturday

225 g (8 oz) boiled new potatoes
Green beans and Tomato Sauce★
100 g (3½ oz) baked salmon
Peach Brûlée
2 glasses dry white wine
Vegetarian option: Spinach Squares★
225 g (8 oz) boiled new potatoes
Green beans and Tomato Sauce★
Peach Brûlée
2 glasses dry white wine

Sunday

75 g (3 oz) Bean Pâté★
2 pitta bread with green salad
grapes
50 g (2 oz) milk chocolate

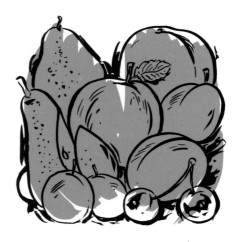

Perfecting Your Lifestyle

There's more to health than just diet. To be most effective Eat for Life Diet has to be part of a healthy lifestyle.

~ The question of drink ~

To start with, there's the question of drink. You don't need alcohol for a healthy diet, but the majority of people 'enjoy a drink'. Despite alcohol being virtually a drug, it is an accepted, even entrenched, part of the work and social scene. To suggest that it may become as unacceptable as smoking would cause outrage.

At any rate, an aperitif has a 'medicinal' purpose. It stimulates the appetite by promoting the secretion of gastric juices and saliva. And as every one knows, good food and wine complement each other. In fact, that's the key to the healthy Mediterranean approach to drinking: wine is mainly taken with food, and in moderation.

While wine can be part of the healthiest diets in the world, the World Health Organisation (WHO) report recommends that we take no more than 4 per cent of our calories as alcohol. And the British goverment's Dietary Reference Values (DRVs) also advise moderation in alcohol intake. Further more, the WHO report comments that where alcohol is not an established social behaviour, people shouldn't start drinking.

There are suggestions that beneficial effects may occur at low levels of alcohol consumption, around 10–20 g (^{1}/3–^{2}/3 oz) of alcohol a day. (This is about 1–1^1/2 units of alcohol – a unit being the amount of alcohol contained in a glass of wine or just under one pint of beer.) It is suggested that people who drink that much may have a reduced risk of heart disease and cholesterol gallstone formation, but most of the evidence does not support this theory.

SOBERING THOUGHTS

The message, if you drink, is to keep within sensible limits and don't overdo it because regular or heavy drinking can lead to serious health problems such as high blood pressure (and stroke), liver cirrhosis, alcoholic brain damage and various cancers. To say nothing of the unpleasant social and emotional consequences of too much alcohol.

~ How much is safe? ~

There's a different answer to that question for men and women. The limit is lower for women because they are less able to metabolise the alcohol, so the liver takes the brunt of the alcohol assault. This means that alcohol stays longer in women's bodies and is more concentrated. Women become drunk faster than men drinking the same amount of alcohol, and they feel the effects for longer. There is also evidence that men have better mechanisms in the stomach for 'diluting' the effects of alcohol, although it is mostly dealt with in the liver.

~ Vitamin gobblers ~

A small amount of alcohol occurs naturally as part of fermentation of fruit juices and other foods, so the body is equipped to deal with alcohol, producing enzymes that detoxify it. However, the process can leave you deficient in minerals and vitamins such as B vitamins and vitamin C.

Vitamin C is at a premium because the liver needs it to produce the enzyme, alcohol dehydrogenase, that converts alcohol to acetaldehyde – too much of which is toxic – and then to non-toxic acetic acid. Vitamin C and the B vitamin thiamin protect against acetaldehyde build-up.

Unfortunately for drinkers, alcohol does not come complete with the vitamins and minerals needed by the body to detoxify it. And because it is a diuretic (which means it stimulates urination), it further depletes vitamin status by increasing losses of vitamins B and C, which are water-soluble.

Unless the diet is rich in nutrient-dense foods, you could be left short of vitamins needed to protect against catching cold or to maintain immunity to other illnesses and disease. Like sugar, the only thing alcohol offers as food is calories. So not only will it go to your head, but also to your waistline.

~ Strong brews ~

The strength of alcoholic drinks varies a lot. For example, beer contains on average 4 per cent alcohol and wines between 7 per

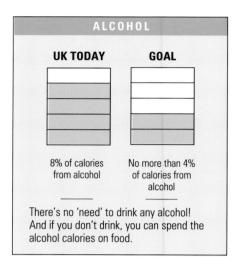

ALCOHOL

UK TODAY	GOAL
8% of calories from alcohol	No more than 4% of calories from alcohol

There's no 'need' to drink any alcohol! And if you don't drink, you can spend the alcohol calories on food.

SPREAD THE LOAD

Even if you don't drink much, the advice is to avoid drinking it all at once. Space out your drinks so that you have one or two alcohol-free days each week. And when drinking, spread out the drinks during a session, interspersing them with non-alcoholic drinks.

cent and 15 per cent. Fortified wines and aperitifs are between 15 per cent and 27 per cent and whisky, gin and other spirits 40 per cent or 70 per cent. The strength by volume of alcohol is on the label, expressed as percentages. However, from a consumer's point of view it's easier to think in terms of alcoholic units. 'Safe' levels have been set for drinking:

- not more than 21 units of alcohol a week for men
- not more than 14 units of alcohol a week for women.

As a general rule one unit of alcohol equals the following:

- 1 single pub measure* ($1/6$th gill) of spirits, or 25 ml (1 fl oz)
- 1 small glass of sherry or other fortified wine, or 79 ml ($2^3/4$ oz)
- 1 small glass of wine, or 125 ml (4 fl oz)
- $1/2$ pint ordinary beer, lager or cider, or 300 ml (10 fl oz)
- $1/4$ pint strong beer, lager or cider, or 125 ml (5 fl oz)
- 2 small glasses of low alcohol wine, or 250 ml (8 fl oz)
- $1^1/2$ pints low alcohol beer, lager or cider, or 900 ml (30 fl oz)

*Scottish pub spirit measures are 1.2 units

The table given here is useful as a general guide but it can be misleading because some wines, beers and spirits are stronger than others. If you enjoy arithmetic you can work out for yourself exactly how many units are in a drink from the alcohol percentage on the label.

For example, a bottle of table wine such as a claret is around 12 per cent alcohol by volume. To work out how many units of alcohol are in the bottle do the following sum:

$$12/1000 \times 750 \text{ ml (the amount in the bottle)} = 9 \text{ units}$$

As there are six, 125 ml (4 oz) glasses of wine in a 750 ml ($1^1/4$ pint) bottle of wine, there are 1.5 units per glass. A lower-strength wine such as some Italian and German white wines, with around 9 per cent alcohol, equals just one unit per glass.

Beers also vary in strength. A pint of ordinary beer contains two units, but a single 440 ml ($3/4$ pint) can of extra strong lager contains four units.

~ Low- and no-alcohol drinks ~

There is no alcohol, or at least not more than 0.05 per cent in alcohol-free drinks. This is the amount that occurs naturally in some fruit juices.

TIME, GENTLEMEN, PLEASE

It takes about an hour for the body to burn one unit of alcohol. A pint of beer and a couple of glasses of wine at lunchtime will still be in the system after work. Seven pints of beer in the evening could mean you are still over the legal driving limit the following morning.

HAIR-OF-THE-DOG

Upset stomachs that accompany hangovers are caused by the acidity of drinks. The only cure for a hangover is plenty of water to drink, possibly some vitamin C, (although this might irritate an upset stomach), rest and something light to eat. Hangover 'cures' don't work. A hair-of-the-dog is dangerous, and black coffee is not particularly helpful because coffee is also a diuretic. Another effect of too much alcohol is low blood sugar. This is because alcohol stimulates production of insulin, which reduces blood sugar levels, leaving you feeling drowsy, weak, wobbly, hungry and even faint.

There is up to 1.2 per cent alcohol in low-alcohol drinks. If you are driving and therefore sticking to low-alcohol drinks, don't assume you can drink an unlimited amount. A small can of low-alcohol beer could contain 0.3 units or about one-third of a unit.

If you have been drinking standard alcoholic drinks earlier, a few low-alcohol drinks could push you over the limit.

~ *Mums-to-be beware* ~

During pregnancy it is best to avoid alcohol, as it can be passed from the mother's bloodstream to the baby and so put the unborn child at risk. There are also suggestions that it is better not to drink (for three months) before conceiving a baby. Even moderate amounts can affect reproduction. One study shows that as little as two pints of beer a day reduces sperm formation.

The greatest risk to babies is during the early weeks of pregnancy, when the baby's brain is developing. But for those who discover they are pregnant and have not given up alcohol, a study by a Scottish team of researchers on pregnant women concluded that there was no adverse effect on babies of mothers-to-be who drank up to eight units per week, in other words one drink a day a day Monday to Saturday and two on Sunday. However, they still advise not to drink when planning to conceive and during a pregnancy.

In America there are government warnings (similar to those on cigarette packs in Britain) on alcoholic drinks, which state: 'Government warning (1) According to the Surgeon General women should not drink alcoholic beverages during pregnancy because of the risk of birth defects (2) Consumption of alcoholic beverages impairs your ability to drive a car or operate machinery, and may cause health problems.'

~ *What about smoking?* ~

Sorry, smokers, it's out. We haven't found anything that allows us to recommend it. The links between smoking and lung cancer and heart disease are incontrovertible. There is also a hazard to 'passive' smokers – those around smokers who inhale sidestream cigarette smoke. There are no health benefits from smoking. The appetite suppressing effect, if any, is far outweighed by the dangers, and surveys show that giving up smoking does not inevitably lead to increased appetite and weight gain.

Smoking makes extra demands for vitamins such as A, C, and E needed by the body to cope with the toxins. Diet surveys show that smokers generally eat fewer nutrient-rich foods, even though their habit makes them need a greater intake of vitamins and minerals.

Giving up smoking is a subject beyond the scope of this book, but if smokers do put on weight after giving up, the Eat for Life Diet will help solve that problem – and help the body recover from the ravages of smoking. For more information contact Quit, 102 Gloucester Place, London W1H 3DA, tel 071 487 2857.

~ *Fun runs and all that* ~

Excercise is a necessary evil for some, and fun for others. There is an impressive list of benefits if you take up aerobic exercise (see table on page 91). By aerobic exercise we mean the type that leaves you breathless and sweaty! The point of this is to exercise the heart which is a muscle and so needs regular exercise to remain 'fit'.

In return for doing between three and five sessions a week for at least 20 to 30 minutes you lose weight, improve your shape, lower your risk of heart disease, reduce fatigue and stress, improve flexibility and reduce the risk of osteoporosis. In short, you will look and feel better. How can you resist? In fact, once you get started, you will wonder why you didn't do it before.

The reason we have to think about exercise and make a positive effort to do something about it is that in most developed countries more importance is placed on desk jobs and sedentary activities than physical ones. So we end up taking less exercise than we need. After a day at the desk, leisure activities can be equally sedentary – watching television and videos, going to the cinema, reading the paper, sitting in the pub or wine bar.

In fact, we are a pretty lazy lot. When we sleep, our basal metabolic rate (the rate at which we burn calories) is 1. As we take so little exercise, during the day for most of us it rises only to 1.4. Sitting at a desk working is 1.1, standing 1.4, walking 3.7, running 8.6. If we take more exercise, we can eat more without getting fat.

So, put this book in a safe place, and take your dog, wife, husband, child, granny . . . for a brisk walk. Seriously, though (as you are still here, reading) try to find an exercise you like and one that fits most easily into your lifestyle.

~ *Sitting comfortably* ~

Building regular exercise into Eat for Life Diet is important. You can maintain the healthy heart and slim figure you have achieved by choosing an aerobic activity, or a selection of different ones, that you can do between three and five times a week for 20 minutes, at a level of 50-80 per cent of your maximum capacity (as measured by taking your pulse, which monitors your heart rate). To discover what your maximum capacity is, subtract your age in years from 220, which gives you the maximum heart rate in beats per minute for your training sessions. To start with, work to 60-70 per cent of your maximum capacity. When fit, you can go to 90 per cent. Measure your heart rate by taking your pulse at your neck or wrist.

If you do a job, such as farming, building, gardening, or sport, that already has a built-in exercise factor (sorry, house work and gardening do not count) you won't need to take exercise sessions. However, for most people their work activity is not enough and is not aerobic. Also, work is often done under stress, which is not a good way to exercise.

Prolonged activity such as the hard physical labour that occupies most people in developing countries seems to be just as good for health as the sporadic bouts of aerobic exercise that are necessary to be healthy and fit in our sedentary Western lifestyles.

If you need further convincing of the benefits of exercise, take a look at the table on page 91.

Or, if you need a starker type of persuasion: don't kid yourself that you will get an early warning before a heart attack, in time to do something about it, (such as taking up exercise or changing your eating habits). You probably won't. Taking sufficient exercise is as beneficial as eating correctly because it improves mood, produces hormones that combat stress, burns calories and tones muscles.

~ The benefits of exercise ~

Physiological functions and capacities that improve with regular exercise are on the left, and the various diseases and conditions that are influenced favourably by these changes are on the right.

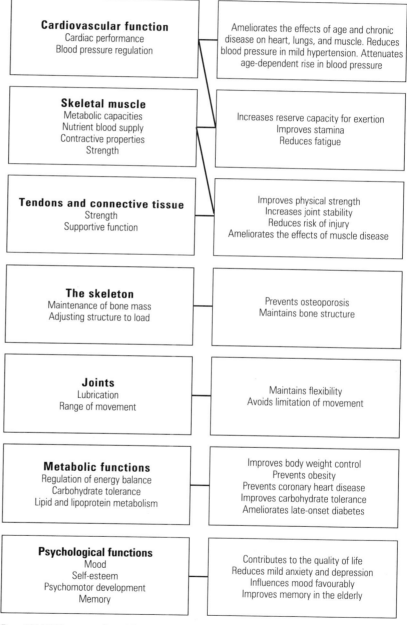

Cardiovascular function
Cardiac performance
Blood pressure regulation

Ameliorates the effects of age and chronic disease on heart, lungs, and muscle. Reduces blood pressure in mild hypertension. Attenuates age-dependent rise in blood pressure

Skeletal muscle
Metabolic capacities
Nutrient blood supply
Contractive properties
Strength

Increases reserve capacity for exertion
Improves stamina
Reduces fatigue

Tendons and connective tissue
Strength
Supportive function

Improves physical strength
Increases joint stability
Reduces risk of injury
Ameliorates the effects of muscle disease

The skeleton
Maintenance of bone mass
Adjusting structure to load

Prevents osteoporosis
Maintains bone structure

Joints
Lubrication
Range of movement

Maintains flexibility
Avoids limitation of movement

Metabolic functions
Regulation of energy balance
Carbohydrate tolerance
Lipid and lipoprotein metabolism

Improves body weight control
Prevents obesity
Prevents coronary heart disease
Improves carbohydrate tolerance
Ameliorates late-onset diabetes

Psychological functions
Mood
Self-esteem
Psychomotor development
Memory

Contributes to the quality of life
Reduces mild anxiety and depression
Influences mood favourably
Improves memory in the elderly

Page 103 WHO report, adapted from Bassey J et al, 'Reasons for advising exercise', *Practitioner* 231:1605-1610 (1987)

~ *How to go about taking more exercise* ~

The main aim of exercise is physical fitness. There are two basic aspects of fitness: stamina and strength. Suppleness is also useful and improves along with the other two.

Before starting any vigorous exercise routine, check with your doctor or instructor if you suspect you have any problem. The best way to begin is to join an exercise class or club where there are supervised activities. If that's not possible, try to find a book or video tape to follow, but make sure it is made by a qualified instructor. The classes and routines should contain the following elements.

Warm-up

A warm-up, usually of five minutes or more, is essential so that you don't damage yourself. Usually it consists of head rolls (rolling the head gently from side to side), arm swings, trunk twists, side bends, marching on the spot and a general warming up of the muscles.

Stamina

To build stamina the warm-up is generally followed by a 20-minute aerobic session, which might be jogging, step or stair climbing or, if you are doing it yourself, your favourite aerobic sport such as swimming. A good starting point for beginners is a low-impact aerobic exercise routine from a book or tape. Often classes are best as they are supervised so you will be stopped if you are doing something wrong, and thus avoid injuries. The atmosphere and enthusiasm of the class also make the whole business easier.

Strength

To build strength you could follow your aerobic session with some press-ups and tummy and leg exercises, which is usual at aerobics classes. Or take yourself off to a gym for a more sophisticated and personally tailored work-out. Ensure that instructors show you how to use the equipment and work out for you a circuit or weight-training programme.

Cool-down

Don't forget to cool down – it prevents aching muscles. A cool-down is a series of stretching exercises, similar to the warm-up. Never stop suddenly, even if it's all too much: you have to keep moving, even if it's fairly gently.

T *A Diet
You Can
Share*

he Eat for Life Diet caters for you, your family and even your friends. If you follow its suggestions and helpful, at-a-glance Eating Plans you can entertain at home with everything from barbecues to Sunday lunch and enjoy eating out in restaurants as well.

~ *Menus for entertaining* ~

Vegetarian Meal

Vegetable Curry (page 124)
Basmati rice (boiled)
Dhal (page 121)
Raita (page 142)
Sliced tomatoes
Pappads

Dried Fruit Salad (page 136) with Almond Biscuits (page 134)

Barbecue

Mushroom à la Grecque (page 122)
Pitta bread

Mexican Beans and Rice (page 110)
West Indian Pork (page 146)
Mango and Tomato Salsa (page 143)
Carrot and Nut Salad (page 130)
Garden Salad (page 130)
Sliced tomatoes

Fresh Fruit Platter (page 135) with Raspberry Sauce (page 140)

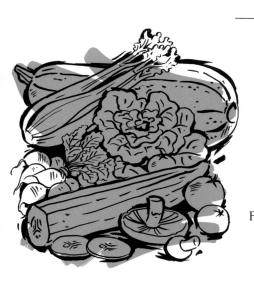

——————————— **Dinner Party 1** ———————————

Tom Yam Gung (Thai fish soup) (page 145)

Venison Ragout (page 146)
Green Beans with Almonds (page 125)
Mixed steamed vegetables
(Mange tout, carrots, baby sweetcorn)
Boiled new potatoes

Simple Trifle (page 137)

——————————— **Dinner Party 2** ———————————

Brushetta (page 104)

Seafood Risotto (page 108)
Large mixed salad (lettuce, tomatoes, radish, cucumber, carrots)

Peaches Stuffed with Almonds (page 137)

~ *Spread the word* ~

You might want to share the Eat for Life Diet philosophy with your family and friends. They too could spend less time in doctors' surgeries if, like you, they adopt the Eat for Life Diet principle of taking responsibility for their own health. All they have to do is:

* follow the Eating Plans or 28-day Slimming Plan if they need to lose weight
* take up exercise and give up smoking
* learn to manage their working hours to avoid too much stress and to make more time for improving relationships with family and friends.

~ *All party dinner party conversation* ~

We're not suggesting you bring politics into this at your next dinner party – far from being healthy, it could simply raise temperatures and blood pressures and give everyone indigestion! Increased public awareness will make eating a healthy diet more widespread, so all of us need to start asking questions. For example, why is it that the UK has seen only a 10 per cent fall in deaths from heart disease among men during the last 20 years and an even worse record of a decline of 2 per cent among women? Why is it that the UK is still at the top of the world table for deaths from heart disease? Why is it that the UK has one of the highest rates of breast and large bowel cancer? Why is it that more than half of middle-aged people are overweight?

It's a complicated set of questions, but you and your friends can make a contribution to change by demanding that the government (of whatever political colour) meet WHO recommendations. Voice your concern about the underlying issues (set out here) to those in authority, such as your local councillors and your MP and MEP.

~ The crucial issue ~

1 Isn't it time we had a national body on food that involves government, the food industry and consumers, with the Department of Health taking the lead?

2 Shouldn't we have the kind of Freedom of Information that is available to consumers in the United States where food manufacturers cannot hide facts about ingredients in our food and drink behind commercial secrecy clauses?

3 Shouldn't the food industry, from supermarkets to the giant food manufacturers, be doing more to improve the nutritional profiles of food products?

4 Isn't it time to end subsidies for butter and meat? If reward is due, surely it should go to production of lower-fat livestock, of fruit and vegetables or of CC foods. Also, let's improve the marketing of fruit and vegetables.

5 Shouldn't nutritional standards for meals in schools and hospitals be introduced on a national basis?

6 Isn't it time that consumer consultation was build into food and health policy?

7 Wouldn't you like to see a concerted effort made to promote education about healthy eating and lifestyle in education establishments, institutions and the community at large?

8 As consumers shouldn't we insist on better nutritional food labelling by provision of simple graphics on the labels? That way it would be possible to make an informed choice about the food we are eating and to follow healthy eating advice and Eat for Life Diet goals.

9 Isn't it time we also had better controls on advertising of junk food to children, health claims on foods, and misleading packaging and advertisements?

10 Shouldn't we try to stop the promotion of Western diets to developing countries at the expense of their traditional healthier foods and diets? And shouldn't we call a halt to the hand outs that give less well-off people at home and abroad the unhealthy surpluses of butter, beef and other saturated fat mountains?

~ *Summing up* ~

In brief, if you want to tell your friends what the Eat for Life Diet is about, its main messages are:

- Eat lots of CC foods like cereals, breads, potatoes, rice and other grains. About half the calorie intake should be from complex carbohydrate foods.
- Eat lots of fruit and vegetables. Aim for at least five portions a day, which adds up to 400 g (14 oz), especially green and yellow fruit and vegetables and citrus fruit.
- Eat the rest of your diet as small amounts of lean meat or low-fat dairy produce or fish or beans. Make a meal of fish instead of meat twice a week; however, animal products are optional and a matter for personal choice.
- Go easy on the alcohol, salt and sugar.
- Go easy on pickled, smoked and salt-preserved foods.

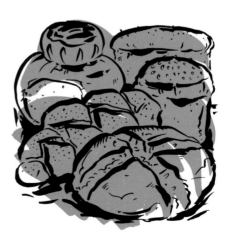

Eat for Life Diet Recipes

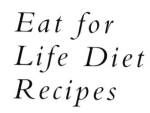

Use these recipes to help you adopt the Eat for Life Diet approach to slimming and healthy eating. The recipes are grouped according to CC foods, on which you should base your meal. Slimmers use these recipes with both the 28-day Slimming Plan and the Easy Option Slimming Plan. They also fit into the Everyday Eating Plan and can be used for entertaining.

~ Putting Eat for Life Diet into your own recipes ~

- Swap lard, dripping, butter and ghee for vegetable oils or margarines that are high in polyunsaturates.
- Use the minimum amount of fat in recipes and when cooking. Keep frying to a minimum; instead bake, steam, boil, poach, grill, dry roast or microwave.
- Don't have too many pastry and pie dishes.
- Swap full fat milk in recipes for skimmed milk.
- Replace cream, cream cheese and other full-fat soft cheeses with fromage frais or other low-fat soft cheeses and different types of yogurt.
- Flavour cottage cheese or other low-fat cheeses with garlic and herbs instead of using standard full fat flavoured creamy cheeses.
- Use only a little hard cheese, because it is very high in fat. Full-flavoured mature Cheddar-style makes a little go a long way. Other tasty cheeses that have a lot of flavour are Gruyère, Emmenthal, Parmesan.
- Cut off all visible fat on meat and use only lean meat. Don't use sausagemeat, luncheon meats, fatty salamis, sausages, meat pies, pâtés, standard mince – or use them only rarely.

COOKING FAT PROFILES			
	Saturated g/100g	Mono-unsaturated g/100g	Polyun-saturated g/100g
Beef dripping	43	48	4
Butter	49	26	2
Coconut oil	85	7	2
Corn oil	17	29	49
Lard	42	42	9
Olive oil	14	70	11
Peanut oil	45	42	8
Polyunsaturate margarine	19	16	60
Safflower seed oil	19	48	28
Soyabean oil	10	13	72
Sunflower seed oil	14	24	57
Wheatgerm oil	14	11	45

- If you make soups, casseroles, stocks etc, skim off any fat before serving. Preferably make them the day before allow them to become completely cold for thorough fat removal.
- Cut down on the amount of salt in cooking and recipes. Spices, herbs and lemon and lime juice give flavour.
- Stock cubes are very salty. Make your own stock, or use low-salt stock cubes.
- Go easy on the soy sauce, barbecue sauce and other high salt sauces.
- In general, cut down on fatty sauces with food. Instead of gravy made with fat from the joint, serve meat with the juices from the meat or a little stock.
- Don't make regular use of creamed and desiccated coconut – it is very high in saturated fat.

FATS IN MEAT			
PERCENTAGE FATTY ACIDS			
	Saturated	Mono-unsaturated	Polyun-saturated
Beef, sirloin, for roasting	45	49	4
Lamb, leg, for roasting	52	41	5
Pork, leg, for roasting	43	48	8
Chicken, roast, meat and skin	35	48	15
Turkey, roast, meat only	37	27	30
Bacon, back, grilled	43	48	8
Liver, lamb's, fried	42	35	18

~ Three steps to healthier cooking and eating ~

Step 1
- Grill food whenever possible.
- Replace white or brown bread with wholemeal as your principle type of bread.
- Cut out sugar in drinks.
- Choose fruit juice or water instead of sugary drinks.
- Use skimmed or semi-skimmed milk instead of whole milk, and yogurt instead of cream.
- Use oils and spreads rich in polyunsaturates.
- Choose lean meat, poultry and fish.

Step 2
- Start to cut down on the overall amount of fat you use in cooking. Replace rice, pasta and breakfast cereals with whole-meal varieties.
- Cut down on between-meal sugar snacks like cakes, biscuits, sweets and chocolates. Snack instead on bread, and fruit.
- Increase the amount of fruit and vegetables you eat, aiming for fresh vegetables and/or a salad daily.

Step 3

- Eat more beans and pulses such as lentils, beans, chickpeas.
- Cut down on the amount of fatty meat you eat, particularly processed meats such as sausages, hamburgers, pâté.
- Make sure the portions of meat and fish you eat are not too large.
- Cut down on the amount of fatty cheeses you eat.
- Try to reduce the amount of salt added during cooking and at the table.
- Try to keep within the recommended limit (see pages 86–87) when drinking alcohol.

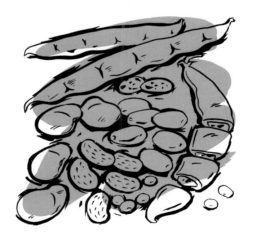

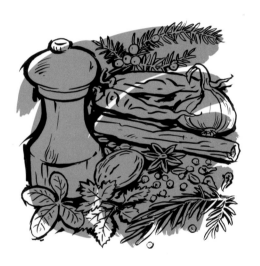

~ *The recipes* ~

SANDWICHES AND FILLINGS

MEXICAN TUNA FILLING

SERVES 2

175 g (6 oz) canned tuna fish

1/4 green pepper, deseeded and chopped

50 g (2 oz) cooked sweetcorn

100 g (3 1/2 oz) cooked kidney beans

dash of Tabasco sauce (optional)

Mix tuna, pepper, sweetcorn, kidney beans and Tabasco sauce together in a bowl.

167 Kcal/701 KJ • 26.8 g Protein • 9.2 g Carbohydrate of which: sugars 2.9 g • 2.7 g Fat of which: saturates 0.1 g • 0.2 g Sodium • 1.7 g Dietary Fibre

SMOKED MACKEREL PATÉ

SERVES 2

100 g (3 1/2 oz) smoked mackerel

50 g (2 oz) low fat curd cheese

1/2 lemon – squeezed

Remove the skin and bones from the smoked mackerel. Place in a liquidiser with cheese and lemon.

149 Kcal/621 KJ • 15.1 g Protein • 1.1 g Carbohydrate of which: sugars 1.1 g • 9.3 g Fat of which: saturates 3.4 g • 0.5 g Sodium • no Dietary Fibre

EGG AND WATERCRESS FILLING

SERVES 1

1 egg, hard boiled

25 g (1 oz) watercress, finely chopped

2 tsp (10 ml) low calorie mayonaise

Chop the hard boiled egg and mix with the watercress and mayonnaise.

125 Kcal/522 KJ • 9.2 g Protein • 1.2 g Carbohydrate of which: 0.8 sugars • 9.4 g Fat of which: 1.9 g saturates • 0.2 g Sodium • 1.7 g Dietary Fibre

NIÇOISE FILLING

SERVES 2

1 egg, hard boiled

75 g (3 oz) canned tuna fish

5 slices red pepper, chopped

3 black olives, chopped

2 tsp (10 ml) low calorie mayonaise

1/2 tsp wine vinegar

Chop the hard boiled egg and mix with the tuna, pepper, olives, mayonnaise and vinegar in a bowl.

124 Kcal/516 KJ • 14.5 g Protein • 1.0 g Carbohydrate of which: sugars 0.7 g • 6.9 g Fat of which: saturates 1.2 g • 0.8 g Sodium • 0.9 Dietary Fibre

PRAWN AND CABBAGE FILLING

SERVES 2

100 g (3¹/₂ oz) prawns
100 g (3¹/₂ oz) white cabbage, finely shredded
15 ml (1 tbsp) lemon juice
10 ml (2 tsp) low calorie mayonnaise

Mix together prawns, cabbage, lemon juice and mayonnaise.

80 Kcal/334 KJ • 12.4 g Protein • 2.5 g Carbohydrate of which: sugars 2.3 g • 2.3 g Fat of which: saturates 0.1 g • 0.9 g Sodium • 1.4 g Dietary Fibre

CHICKEN AND BLUE CHEESE SALAD TOASTED SANDWICH

SERVES 2

75 g (3 oz) roasted chicken
50 g (2 oz) dolcelatte, grated
4 large thick slices wholemeal bread
10 ml (2 tsp) low fat spread
1 sliced tomato
lettuce

Thinly slice the chicken. Toast the bread and spread with the low fat spread. Place the salad, cheese and chicken mixture evenly between the bread.

182 Kcal/763 KJ • 12.1 g Protein • 17.1 g Carbohydrate of which: sugars 1.9 g • 7.7 g Fat of which: saturates 3.8 g • 0.3 g Sodium • 2.5 g Dietary Fibre

TABOULLEH

SERVES 2

50 g (2 oz) burghul or cracked wheat
large chuck of cucumber
¹/₃ green pepper deseeded and finely diced
small red onion, diced
30ml (2 tbsp) freshly chopped mint
juice of ¹/₂ lemon
black pepper

Cook the wheat in twice its volume of boiling water for 10 minutes, or leave it to stand in the same amount of just boiled water for 15 minutes until the grain has swelled and softened. Drain and squeeze out moisture and place the wheat in a bowl. Stir in the remaining ingredients.

103 Kcal/431 KJ • 3.2 g Protein • 22g Carbohydrate of which: sugar 2.8 g • 0.6 Fat of which: saturates trace • trace Sodium • 0.7 g Dietary Fibre

CHICKEN AND TABOULLEH SANDWICH

SERVES 1

2 slices wholemeal bread
7 g (¹/₄ oz) low fat spread
50 g (2 oz) lean roast chicken
30 ml (2 tbsp) taboulleh (see above)

Thinly spread the bread with the spread. Place chicken and taboulleh on one slice of bread, top with the second slice.

373 Kcal/1574 KJ • 24.2 g Protein • 54.8 g Carbohydrate, of which: 3.3 g sugars • 7.8 g Fat of which: 1.5 g saturates • 0.7 g Sodium • 6.8 g Dietary Fibre

CRAB STUFFED PITTA BREAD

SERVES 1

60 g (2¹/₂ oz) white crab meat
50 g (2 oz) white cabbage, finely chopped
1 tsp (5 ml) lemon juice
1 tsp (5 ml) low calorie mayonnaise
1 large wholemeal pitta bread

Mix the cabbage, lemon juice and mayonnaise together in a bowl. Put the mixture inside the pitta bread, then top with the crab meat.

390 Kcal/1645 KJ • 22.0 g Protein • 57.0 g Carbohydrate, of which: 4.2 g sugars • 9.9 g Fat, of which: 1.2 g saturates • 0.7 g Sodium • 9.9 g Dietary Fibre

BRUSHETTA

SERVES 2

8 cherry tomatoes, cut in half
2 thick slices ciabatta bread
2 tbsp (30 ml) black olive pâté
freshly chopped basil

Grill the tomatoes under a hot grill. At the same time toast the bread and spread one side with the olive paste. Top with the tomatoes and basil.

170 Kcal/709 KJ • 5.6 g Protein • 26.4 g Carbohydrates, of which: sugars 3.7 g • 5.4 g Fat of which: saturates 0.8 g • 0.7 g Sodium • 4.6 g Dietary Fibre

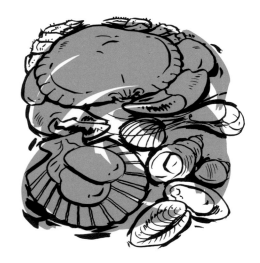

POTATOES

SUMMER SOUP

SERVES 4

750 ml (1¼ pints) chicken or vegetable stock

350 g (12 oz) potatoes, scrubbed and cut into large pieces

1 large onion, peeled and chopped

2 leeks, well rinsed and sliced

10 ml (2 tsp) olive oil

50 g (2 oz) basil leaves, chopped

100 g (3½ oz) watercress

ground black pepper

Combine the stock, potatoes and onion in a large saucepan. Cook until the potatoes are tender (about 20 minutes). Heat oil in a non stick fry pan and sauté leeks for 10 minutes until almost tender. Add the basil and watercress and cook for a further 5 minutes. Purée the soup in the blender. Add black pepper. Return to the pan and heat gently.

137 Kcal/572 KJ • 5.1 g Protein • 24.9 g Carbohydrate, of which: 6.9 g sugars • 2.7 g Fat, of which: 0.4 g saturates • 0.2 g Sodium • 6.4 g Dietary Fibre

INDIAN POTATOES

SERVES 4

450 g (1 lb) potatoes, scrubbed and chopped into small pieces

1 cauliflower, chopped into small florets

10 ml (2 tsp) oil

5 ml (1 tsp) turmeric

2.5 ml (½ tsp) cumin seeds

ground black pepper

100 g (3½ oz) mushrooms

Par-boil the potatoes for 5 minutes, then add the cauliflower and cook for a further 4 minutes. Drain. Heat oil in a wok and then add the spices. Cook for about 1 minute and then add the vegetables. Cook for 5 minutes or until the vegetables are tender.

128 Kcal (534 Kj) • 3.9 g Protein • 23.4 g Carbohydrate, of which: 1.4 g sugars • 2.8 g Fat, of which: 0.4 g saturates • trace Sodium • 3.8 g Dietary Fibre

TUNA AND POTATO BAKE

SERVES 4

350 g (12 oz) onion, peeled and sliced

1 clove garlic, crushed

5 ml (1 tsp) sunflower oil

400 g (14 oz) chopped canned tomatoes

15 ml (1 tbsp) tomato purée

200 g (7 oz) canned tuna, drained

12 black olives, chopped

pinch mixed herbs

2.5 ml (½ tsp) sugar

350 g (12 oz) potatoes, scrubbed and cooked

25 g (1 oz) breadcrumbs

Soften onion and garlic in oil in a non stick frypan. Add tomatoes and tomato purée and simmer for about 10 minutes. Add tuna, black olives, herbs and sugar and cook for a further 5 minutes. Meanwhile heat the oven to 190°C, 375°F mark 5. Grease an ovenproof dish and add potatoes and sauce ending with a layer of sauce. Sprinkle with breadcrumbs and cook for 40 minutes.

217 Kcal/908 KJ • 18.2 g Protein • 30.7 g Carbohydrate, of which: 8.8 g sugars • 3.2 g Fat, of which: 0.4 g saturates • 0.2 g sodium • 5.3 g Dietary Fibre

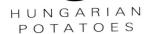

HUNGARIAN POTATOES

SERVES 4

10 ml (2 tsp) olive oil
1 large onion, peeled and chopped
2 cloves garlic, crushed
1 large aubergine, diced
2 red peppers, deseeded and sliced
15 ml (1 tbsp) paprika
100 g (4 oz) mushrooms, sliced
400 g (14 oz) chopped canned tomatoes
45 ml (3 tbsp) tomato purée
sprig of thyme
350 g (12 oz) potatoes, scrubbed and cooked until just tender
ground black pepper
30 ml (2 tbsp) water

Heat oil in a large casserole dish. Add the onion and cook over a low heat for 10 minutes or until brown. Add garlic and cook for a further 2 minutes. Add the aubergine and pepper, cover with a lid and cook for a further 5 minutes. Add the paprika and cook for 2 minutes. Mix in the remaining vegetables, tomato purée, thyme and 2 tablespoons water and simmer for 45 – 60 minutes or until cooked.

159 Kcal/667 KJ • 5.6 g Protein • 3.2 g Carbohydrate of which: sugars 0.4 g • 29.1 g Fat of which: saturates 10.8 g • trace Sodium • 6.3 g Dietary Fibre

Variations: Chick Pea Hot Pot. Delete the potatoes from the above recipe and add 14 oz (400 g) cooked chick peas instead. Add 1 tsp ground cinnamon as well as the other seasoning.

184 Kcal/771 KJ • 11.4 g Protein • 3.5 g Fat of which: saturates 0.4 g • 29 g Carbohydrate of which: sugars 11.9 g • trace Sodium • 10.5 g Dietary Fibre

Ratatouille. Delete the potatoes and mushrooms from the above recipe and add 1 lb (450 g) sliced courgettes at the same time as the aubergine. Delete the paprika.

117 Kcal/492 KJ • 6.1 g Protein • 3.6 g Fat of which: saturates 0.4 g • 17.0 g Carbohydrate of which: sugars 10.4 g • trace Sodium • 5.5 g Dietary Fibre

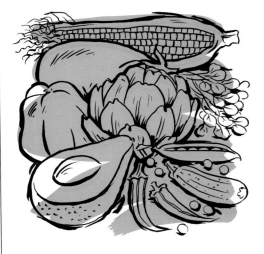

RICE

ARROZ VERDE

SERVES 4

5 ml (1 tsp) sunflower oil
2 green peppers, deseeded and chopped
1/2 onion, peeled and finely chopped
1 green chilli, deseeded and finely chopped or pinch chilli powder
60 ml (4 tbsp) chopped fresh parsley
225 g (8 oz) long grain white rice
600 ml (1 pint) vegetable stock
ground black pepper

Heat the oil in a large saucepan and fry the peppers, onion and chilli for 5 minutes. Add the remaining ingredients, bring to the boil, cover and simmer for 12 minutes or until the rice is tender.

240 Kcal/1005 KJ • 5.8 g Protein • 48.2 g Carbohydrate, of which: 3.1 g sugars • 2.4 g Fat, of which: 0.3 g saturates • 0.2 g Sodium • 1.0 g Dietary Fibre

SPICY RICE

SERVES 4

225 g (8 oz) long grain brown rice
5 ml (1 tsp) ground turmeric
1 stick cinnamon
1 bay leaf
4 green cardamon pods
6 black peppercorns

Put all the ingredients in a saucepan with enough water and bring to the boil. Cook for 35 minutes or until the rice is tender. Drain and serve.

205 Kcal/872 KJ • 3.9 g Protein • 46.5 g Carbohydrate, of which: 0.7 g sugars • 1.7 g Fat, of which: no saturates trace Sodium • 2.1 g Dietary Fibre

NASI GORENG (WITH CHICKEN OR EGG)

SERVES 4

10 ml (2 tsp) sunflower oil
4 small chicken breasts
2 large onions, peeled and chopped
3 cloves garlic, crushed
1.25 ml (1/4 tsp) chilli powder
1.25 ml (1/4 tsp) laos (optional)
10 ml (2 tsp) ground cumin
5 ml (1 tsp) ground coriander
30 ml (2 tbsp) soy sauce
15 ml (1 tbsp) tomato ketchup
275 g (10 oz) long grain brown rice, cooked

Heat the oil in a large non stick pan and cook the chicken breasts for about 15 – 20 minutes. Remove the chicken and allow to cool. Add the onions to the pan and cook for 15 minutes until well browned. Add the garlic and cook for a further 1 minute. Stir in the spices and cook for 2 minutes. Cut the chicken breasts into small pieces and add to the pan with the soy sauce, tomato ketchup and brown rice. Cover and cook for 20 minutes, stirring frequently. Add 15 – 30 ml (1 – 2 tbsp) water if necessary.

267 Kcal/1117 KJ • 24.9 g Protein • 28.3 g Carbohydrate, of which: 4.7 g sugars • 6.7 g Fat, of which: 1.4 g saturates • 0.1 g Sodium • 1.8 g Dietary Fibre

Variation: Egg Nasi Goreng. Instead of using chicken, make the nasi goreng with an omelette. Make a flat omelette with 4 eggs. When cooked, cut into strips and add 5 minutes before serving. If all the family aren't vegetarian, separate the dish into the appropriate portions after cooking the spices. Add the chicken to the portion for meat eaters and later add the omelette to the other portion.

265 Kcal/1109 KJ • 9.6 g Protein • 28.3 g Carbohydrate, of which: 4.7 g sugars • 13.4 g Fat, of which: 4.8 g saturates • 0.7 g Sodium • 1.8 g Dietary Fibre

SEAFOOD RISOTTO

SERVES 4

10 ml (2 tsp) sunflower oil

1 large onion, peeled and chopped

2 cloves garlic, crushed

275 g (10 oz) American long grain rice

150 ml (1/4 pint) dry white wine

450 ml (3/4 pint) vegetable stock

150 g (5 oz) prepared squid, chopped

225 g (8 oz) peeled prawns

1 red pepper, deseeded and chopped

1 large courgette, sliced

1 large pinch chilli powder

90 ml (6 tbsp) chopped fresh mixed herbs such as basil, coriander and parsley

Heat the oil in a large heavy casserole and slowly cook the onion for 10 minutes. Add the garlic and rice and cook for a further 4 minutes. Add the wine and simmer until most of the liquid is absorbed. Stir in half of the stock and simmer until the liquid is absorbed, stirring frequently. Add the remainder of the stock and simmer until the liquid is absorbed. Mix in the fish, cover and cook for 5 minutes. Stir in the vegetables and chilli powder, cover and cook for a further 7 minutes. Add more water if the risotto starts to dry out. Finally add the herbs, stir and then serve.

389 Kcal/1647 KJ • 16.3 g Protein • 65.5 g Carbohydrate, of which: 5.1 g sugars • 6.2 g Fat, of which: 0.4 g saturates • 0.4 g Sodium • 3.2 g Dietary Fibre

BROWN RICE SALAD

SERVES 4

225 g (8 oz) long grain brown rice, cooked

150 g (5 oz) French beans, trimmed

75 g (3 oz) sweetcorn, cooked

1/2 red pepper, deseeded and chopped

75 g (3 oz) seedless grapes

3 spring onions, chopped

350 g (12 oz) cooked chicken, cubed (optional)

30 ml (2 tbsp) French dressing (see page 144)

Mix all the ingredients together in a large bowl.

412 Kcal/1736 KJ • 27.1 g Protein • 52.8 g Carbohydrate, of which: 5.5 g sugars • 11.2 g Fat, of which: 2.3 g saturates • 0.2 g Sodium • 4.6 g Dietary Fibre

LEMON RICE WITH CASHEWS

SERVES 4

225 g (8 oz) easy cook brown rice

15 ml (1 tbsp) grated lemon rind

juice of 1 lemon

50 g (2 oz) cashew nuts (not for dieters!)

ground black pepper

Cook the rice in a pan of boiling water until tender, then drain. Add the remaining ingredients and stir over a low heat for 3 minutes for flavours to mix. Serve.

WITHOUT CASHEWS
204 Kcal/867 KJ • 3.9 g Protein • 46.4 g Carbohydrate, of which: 1.4 g sugars • 1.6 g Fat, of which: no saturates • trace Sodium • 3.2 g Dietary Fibre

WITH CASHEWS
274 Kcal/1160 KJ • 6.1 g Protein • 49.9 g Carbohydrate, of which: 1.4 g sugars • 7.3 g Fat, of which: no saturates • trace Sodium • 3.2 g Dietary Fibre

LEEK OR COURGETTE RISOTTO

SERVES 4

10 ml (2 tsp) sunflower oil

1 small onion, peeled and sliced

1 clove garlic, crushed

275 g (10 oz) leeks, washed and sliced, or 350 g (12 oz) courgettes, sliced

350 g (12 oz) risotto rice

1.5 litres (2½ pints) vegetable stock

large handful parsley, chopped

15 ml (1 tbsp) grated Parmesan cheese

Heat the oil in a large saucepan and cook the onion and garlic until soft, about 5 minutes. Add the leeks or courgettes and cook for 7 minutes, stirring frequently. Add the rice and stir a couple of times until it is coated with oil. Stir in the stock, a ladleful at a time, always waiting for the previous addition to be absorbed before adding the next ladleful. Cook the rice for about 20 minutes or until al dente. As soon as the rice is tender, stir in the parsley and Parmesan cheese and serve.

278 Kcal/1159 KJ • 7.4 g Protein • 29.5 g Carbohydrate, of which: 11.0 g sugars • 14.7 g Fat, of which: 1.6 g saturates • 0.4 g Sodium • 4.4 g Dietary Fibre

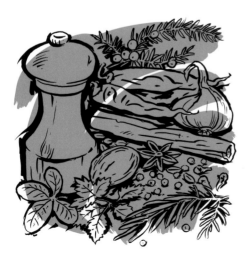

KEDGEREE

SERVES 4

225 g (8 oz) easy cook brown rice

600 ml (1 pint) fish stock

225 g (8 oz) mange tout

400 g (14 oz) salmon

1 bay leaf

6 whole black peppercorns

juice of 1 lemon

ground black pepper

large handful parsley, chopped

2 spring onions, chopped

Cook the rice in the stock. When nearly cooked, add the mange tout and cook for a further 5 minutes. Drain. Meanwhile, place the fish in a frying pan with the bay leaf, peppercorns and the juice from ½ the lemon. Add just enough water to cover the fish and simmer for 15 minutes or until tender. Drain and flake the fish into large chunks, discarding any bones. Mix together the rice, fish, black pepper, remaining lemon juice, parsley and spring onions.

399 Kcal/1682 KJ • 24.3 g Protein • 48.8 g Carbohydrate, of which: 1.4 g sugars • 13.2 g Fat, of which: 2.9 g saturates • 0.1 g Sodium • 8.1 g Dietary Fibre

PERSIAN RICE

SERVES 4

225 g (8 oz) Bastami rice

large handful parsley, chopped

large handful coriander, chopped

handful tarragon, chopped

handful mint, chopped

ground black pepper

Gently cook the rice in a pan of boiling water for 8 minutes, then drain. Return the rice to the pan, add the herbs and black pepper. Cover the pan and leave for 5 minutes without removing the lid. Serve.

202 Kcal/845 KJ • 4.2 g Protein • 44.9 g Carbohydrate, of which: no sugars • 0.3 g Fat, of which: no saturates • no Sodium • no Dietary Fibre

MEXICAN BEANS AND RICE

SERVES 4

10 ml (2 tsp) sunflower oil

1 large onion, peeled and chopped

1 green chilli, deseeded and chopped

225 g (8 oz) long grain rice

2 tomatoes, skinned and deseeded

750 ml (1¼ pint) vegetable stock

100 g (3½ oz) pinto or red kidney beans, cooked

ground black pepper

Heat the oil in a non stick fry pan and cook
the onion until soft, about 5 minutes. Add
the chilli and rice and cook for a further 2
minutes or until the rice turns opaque.
Chop the tomatoes and add to the rice.
Pour in the stock, bring to the boil, cover
and simmer for 10 minutes. Add the beans
and black pepper, adding extra water if
necessary. Cook for a further 5 minutes.
Drain and serve.

*264 Kcal/1120 KJ • 6.8 g Protein • 57.1 g Carbohydrate,
of which: 4.0 g sugars • 2.5 g Fat, of which: 0.4 g saturates
• 0.2 g Sodium • 4.3 g Dietary Fibre*

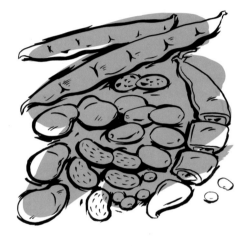

PASTA AND NOODLES

PASTA SALAD

SERVES 4

1 lettuce, washed and dried
450 g (1 lb) cooked wholemeal pasta
225 g (8 oz) sweetcorn
350 g (12 oz) white crab meat
1 apple, cored and diced
2 tomatoes, chopped
1 courgette, sliced
large handful basil, chopped (optional)
60 ml (4 tbsp) French dressing (see page 144)
ground black pepper

Line a salad bowl with the lettuce. Mix together the remaining ingredients and place in the centre of the lettuce lined bowl.

336 Kcal/1409 KJ • 23.9 g Protein • 34.4 g Carbohydrate, of which 12.0 g sugars • 12.4 g Fat, of which: 1.6 g saturates • 0.5 g Sodium • 5.6 g Dietary Fibre

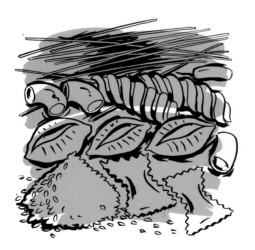

PASTA, BEAN AND VEGETABLE SOUP

SERVES 4

10 ml (2 tsp) olive oil
1 large onion, peeled and chopped
2 carrots, peeled and diced
2 sticks celery, chopped
1 clove garlic, crushed
4 stalks parsley
2 sprigs thyme
1 bay leaf
1 piece lemon rind
225 g (8 oz) white cabbage, finely sliced
100 g (3½ oz) frozen peas
400 g (14 oz) chopped tinned tomatoes
150 g (5 oz) tomato purée
400 g (14 oz) cooked haricot beans
175 g (6 oz) macaroni
2 rashers lean back bacon, cut into small pieces
ground black pepper
450 ml (¾ pint) water

Heat the oil in a large saucepan and cook the onion, carrot and celery until soft, about 8 minutes. Add the garlic and cook for a further 2 minutes. Tie the parsley, thyme, bay leaf and lemon rind together with a piece of string to make a bouquet garni. Add the cabbage, peas, tomatoes, tomato purée, beans, macaroni, bacon, black pepper and bouquet garni to the pan with the water. Bring to the boil and simmer for 20 minutes. Remove the bouquet garni and serve.

411 Kcal/1729 KJ • 20.5 g Protein • 63.6 g Carbohydrate, of which 14.4 g sugars • 10.1 g Fat, of which: 3.0 g saturates • 0.3 g Sodium • 17.3 g Dietary Fibre

PASTA WITH KIDNEY BEANS AND BACON

SERVES 4

10 ml (2 tsp) sunflower oil

1 large onion, peeled and chopped

1 clove garlic, crushed

1.25 ml (1/4 tsp) chilli powder

225 g (8 oz) wholemeal pasta

400 g (14 oz) can kidney beans, drained

400 g (14 oz) can chopped tomatoes

100 g (4 oz) lean bacon, chopped into bite sized pieces

200 g (7 oz) can sweetcorn, drained

7.5 ml (1/2 tbsp) tomato purée

ground black pepper

30 ml (2 tbsp) chopped fresh parsley

Heat oil in a pan and cook the onion for about 8 minutes until soft. Add the garlic and chilli powder and fry for 1 minute. Meanwhile cook the pasta in a large pan of boiling water for 10 minutes or until al dente. Drain. When the onion is softened add the beans, tomatoes, bacon, sweetcorn, tomato purée and black pepper. Simmer for 15 minutes. Mix the pasta with the bean sauce and simmer for 5 minutes. Sprinkle with parsley and serve.

413 Kcal/1740 KJ • 21.5 g Protein • 72.6 g Carbohydrate, of which 11.4 g sugars • 6.1 g Fat, of which: 1.3 g saturates • 0.7 g Sodium • 14.7 g Dietary Fibre

PASTA AI FUNGHI

SERVES 2

150 g (5 oz) shitake mushrooms

150 g (5 oz) oyster mushrooms

100 g (3 1/2 oz) button mushrooms

15 ml (1 tbsp) olive oil

1 small onion, peeled and finely chopped

1 clove garlic, crushed

1/2 green pepper, deseeded and chopped

225 g (8 oz) fresh pasta

30 ml (2 tbsp) chopped fresh coriander

40 g (1 1/2 oz) pumpkin seeds, toasted (optional)

soy sauce, to serve (optional)

Wipe the mushrooms and slice the large ones. Heat the oil in a pan and cook the onion, garlic and pepper until browned and softened, about 5-8 minutes. Add the mushrooms and continue cooking for 5 minutes (the pan will be full at this stage but they will cook down). Cook the pasta in a large pan of boiling water for 7 minutes or until tender. Add enough water to the mushroom mixture to prevent sticking and cook for a further 5 minutes. Stir in the coriander. Serve the mushroom sauce with the freshly cooked pasta. Sprinkle the pumpkin seeds over the sauce, if using, and dress with a small amount of soy sauce if liked. Variations: Instead of pasta, serve the sauce with toasted bread, cooked rice or jacket potato.

427 Kcal/1799 KJ • 16.9 g Protein • 46.2 g Carbohydrate, of which 9.3 g sugars • 20.0 g Fat, of which: 4.5 g saturates • trace Sodium • 10.3 g Dietary Fibre

PASTA WITH GREEN BEANS AND PRAWNS OR MUSHROOMS

SERVES 4

750 g (1 1/2 lb) French beans, trimmed
225 g (8 oz) egg noodles
7.5 ml (1 1/2 tsp) sunflower oil
2.5 ml (1/2 tsp) sesame oil
350 g (12 oz) peeled prawns
2 cloves garlic, crushed
45 ml (3 tbsp) soy sauce

Cut the French beans in half. Bring a large pan of water to the boil and add the beans. Cook for 5 minutes or until just tender. Drain. Meanwhile, cook the egg noodles in a large pan of boiling water for 10 – 12 minutes or according to packet instructions. Drain. Heat the oils in a wok and stir-fry the prawns and garlic for 2 minutes. Add the French beans and noodles and stir for 4 minutes. Sprinkle over the soy sauce.

361 Kcal/1518 KJ • 28.8 g Protein • 44.4 g Carbohydrate, of which 2.6 g sugars • 8.8 Fat, of which: 0.5 g saturates • 1.5 g Sodium • 8.8 g Dietary Fibre

Variation: Pasta with green beans and mushrooms. Use 350 g (12 oz) mushrooms instead of prawns. A mixture of cep and chanterelle mushrooms have a rich flavour but field mushrooms also make a tasty dish. Cook for 5 minutes before adding the noodles and French beans.

278 Kcal/1173 KJ • 10.6 g Protein • 44.4 g Carbohydrate, of which: 2.6 g sugars • 7.7 g Fat, of which: 0.4 g saturates • 0.1 g Sodium • 11.0 g Dietary Fibre

PASTA WITH TOMATO AND AUBERGINE SAUCE

SERVES 4

1 large aubergine, diced
10 ml (2 tsp) olive oil
1 quantity tomato sauce (see page 142)
85 ml (3 fl oz) red wine
4 anchovy fillets, finely chopped
25 g (1 oz) capers (optional)
225 g (8 oz) pasta

Heat the oil in a large saucepan and cook the aubergine for 5 minutes, stirring constantly. Cover and cook over a low heat for another 5 minutes or until soft. Add tomato sauce, wine, anchovy fillets and capers, if using, and simmer for 15 minutes. Meanwhile, cook the pasta in a large pan of boiling water for 10 minutes or until al dente. Drain and mix the sauce with the pasta.

276 Kcal/1166 KJ • 8.8 g Protein • 48.2 g Carbohydrate, of which 6.5 g sugars • 5.1 g Fat, of which: 0.7 g saturates • 0.1 g Sodium • 6.2 g Dietary Fibre

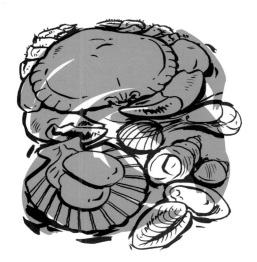

PASTA WITH FRESH TOMATOES

SERVES 4

20 ml (4 tsp) olive oil
10 ml (2 tsp) finely chopped fresh root ginger (optional)
750 g (1¹/₂ lb) canned chopped tomatoes or 1 kg (2 lb) extra-ripe tomatoes, skinned and chopped
5 ml (1 tsp) sugar
ground black pepper
225 g (8 oz) pasta

Heat the oil in large saucepan and gently cook the ginger and tomatoes for 10 minutes, stirring frequently. Add the sugar and black pepper. Cook the pasta in a large pan of boiling water for 10 minutes or until al dente. Drain and serve with the sauce.

273 Kcal/1158 KJ • 8.5 g Protein • 49.4 g Carbohydrate, of which 7.5 g sugars • 6.0 g Fat, of which: 0.9 g saturates • trace Sodium • 5.6 g Dietary Fibre

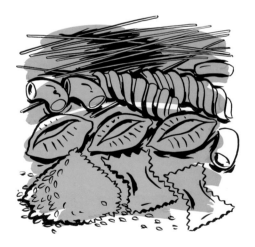

PASTA WITH LIVER

SERVES 4

350 g (12 oz) chicken livers, trimmed
10 ml (2 tsp) sunflower oil
1 large onion, peeled and finely chopped
2 cloves garlic, crushed
2 tomatoes, skinned
150 ml (¹/₄ pint) chicken stock
sprig sage
ground black pepper
450 g (1 lb) fresh pasta

Cut the chicken livers into large pieces. Heat the oil in a large non stick fry pan and cook the onion and garlic until soft, about 5 – 8 minutes. Stir in the tomatoes and cook for a further 4 minutes. Add the chicken stock and simmer for about 10 minutes. Stir in the chicken livers, sage and black pepper and cook over a gentle heat for 25 minutes or until cooked. Keep uncovered if it starts to stick and add a little water, but the mixture should be fairly thick. Meanwhile, cook the pasta in a large pan of boiling water for about 7 minutes. Drain. Mix the sauce with pasta.

364 Kcal/1536 KJ • 25.1 g Protein • 48.6 g Carbohydrate, of which 6.0 g sugars • 9.1 g Fat, of which: 2.2 g saturates • 0.3 g Sodium • 4.3 g Dietary Fibre

SPICY CHICKEN OR NUTTY NOODLES

SERVES 4

225 g (8 oz) noodles
5 ml (1 tsp) sunflower oil
1 large onion, peeled and chopped
2.5 cm (1 inch) piece fresh root ginger, peeled and finely chopped
2 cloves garlic, crushed
15 ml (1 tbsp) curry powder
1 dried red chilli, crushed (optional)
50 ml (2 fl oz) chicken stock
25 ml (1 fl oz) dry sherry
15 ml (1 tbsp) tomato purée
15 ml (1 tbsp) soy sauce
250 g (8 oz) beansprouts
250 g (8 oz) cooked chicken, cut into small pieces

Cook the noodles in a pan of boiling water for 3 minutes. Drain and rinse with cold water. Heat the oil in a wok, and stir-fry the onion and ginger for 4 minutes. Add the garlic, curry powder and chilli, if using, and fry for a further minute. Add the stock, sherry, tomato purée, soy sauce and beansprouts and cook for 4 minutes, stirring frequently. Stir in the chicken and noodles and cook for 4 minutes. Serve.

412 Kcal/1735 KJ • 25.1 g Protein • 51.1 g Carbohydrate, of which 3.1 g sugars • 12.1 g Fat, of which: 1.6 g saturates • 0.2 g Sodium • 3.5 g Dietary Fibre

Variation. Spicy nutty noodles. Use 75 g (3 oz) chopped peanuts instead of the chicken, adding them with the stock.

422 Kcal/1776 KJ • 15.2 g Protein • 52.7 g Carbohydrate, of which 3.7 g sugars • 16.9 g Fat, of which: 1.9 g saturates • 0.1 g Sodium • 5.0 g Dietary Fibre

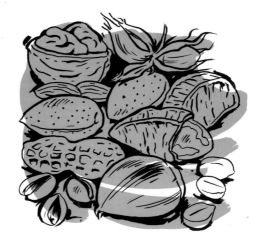

BEANS AND LENTILS

CHICKEN WITH CHICK PEAS AND APRICOTS

SERVES 4

4 large chicken breasts, each cut into 3 pieces
1 dried red chilli
1 small cinnamon stick
5 ml (1 tsp) cumin seeds
4 green cardamom pods
8 cloves
2.5 cm (1 inch) piece fresh root ginger, peeled and finely chopped
2 cloves garlic, crushed
100 g (4 oz) dried no-soak apricots
150 ml (¼ pint) water
10 ml (2 tsp) sunflower oil
1 large onion, peeled and chopped
15 ml (1 tbsp) tomato purée
15 ml (1 tbsp) white malt vinegar
10 ml (2 tsp) sugar
400 g (14 oz) canned chick peas, drained

Place the chicken into a large non-porous bowl. Put the chilli, cinnamon, cumin, cardamom pods and cloves into a spice grinder and grind as fine as possible. Rub half the spice mixture into the chicken with half the ginger and garlic. Set aside for at least 1 hour. Cook the apricots in the water until tender. Leave to cool in the pan. Heat a wok, add the oil and cook the onion for 7 minutes, stirring frequently. Stir in the rest of the ginger and garlic and cook for a further minute. Remove the onion mixture. Add the chicken and cook for 3 minutes until lightly cooked. Add the remaining spice mixture and onion mixture and cook for further 2 minutes. Stir in the tomato purée, vinegar, sugar, chick peas and apricots with the cooking juice. Cook for 15 minutes and serve. Variations: Use 450 g (1 lb) leg of lamb chops instead of chicken. Cook for 30 minutes instead of 15 minutes at the end of cooking. (Alternatively for the spices, mix together a pinch of chilli powder, 2.5 ml (1/2 tsp) ground cinnamon, 5 ml (1 tsp) ground cumin and 2.5 ml (1/2 tsp) garam marsala.

321 Kcal/1339 KJ • 29.9 g Protein • 36.2 g Carbohydrate, of which: 19.3 g sugars • 7.3 g Fat, of which: 1.8 g saturates • 0.1 g Sodium • 11.9 g Dietary Fibre

KEEMA

SERVES 4

350 g (12 oz) lean minced beef
5 ml (1 tsp) sunflower oil
1 large onion, peeled and sliced
1 clove garlic, crushed
5 ml (1 tsp) ground cumin
5 ml (1 tsp) ground turmeric
1.25 ml (¼ tsp) chilli powder
225 g (8 oz) frozen peas
15 ml (1 tbsp) tomato purée

Brown the minced beef in a a large nonstick pan, then remove to a large bowl. Heat the oil in the pan and cook the onion until soft, about 8 minutes. Add the garlic and spices and cook for a further 2 minutes. Return the meat to the pan, add the peas, tomato purée and a little water. Cover and simmer for 25 minutes.

175 Kcal/731 KJ • 22.0 g Protein • 7.7 g Carbohydrate, of which: 4.2 g sugars • 6.5 g Fat, of which: 2.0 g saturates • trace Sodium • 7.6 g Dietary Fibre

BUTTER BEAN AND MUSHROOM BAKE

SERVES 4

225 g (8 oz) dried butter beans, cooked, or 600 g (1 lb 5 oz) canned butter beans
15 ml (1 tbsp) lemon juice
ground black pepper
5 ml (1 tsp) sunflower oil
250 g (8 oz) mushrooms, sliced
25 g (1 oz) sunflower margarine
25 g (1 oz) wholemeal flour
300 ml (1/2 pint) water
25 g (1 oz) Cheddar cheese, grated
25 g (1 oz) fresh breadcrumbs

Soak the dried butter beans for at least 4 hours. Drain and cook in a pan of unsalted boiling water for 40 – 50 minutes or until tender. Drain. If using canned beans, just drain. Put the beans into a large greased ovenproof dish. Add the lemon juice and black pepper. Heat the oil in a pan and fry the mushrooms then add to the dish. Heat the margarine in a non stick saucepan and add the flour. Cook for 2 minutes over a low heat, stirring, then slowly add the water to make a pouring sauce. Pour over the butter beans and mushrooms. Sprinkle with cheese and breadcrumbs. Cook, in the oven at 180°C (350°F) mark 4 for 25 minutes.

275 Kcal/1147 KJ • 14.9 g Protein • 34.6 g Carbohydrate, of which: 2.6 g sugars • 9.6 g Fat, of which: 2.8 g saturates • 0.2 g Sodium • 10.1 g Dietary Fibre

LAZY LENTILS

SERVES 4

175 g (6 oz) red lentils
100 g (3 1/2 oz) Cheddar cheese, grated
5 ml (1 tsp) vegetable extract
5 ml (1 tsp) dried mixed herbs
10 ml (2 tsp) sunflower oil
2 medium onions, peeled and chopped
1 clove garlic, crushed
300 ml (1/2 pint) water

Put the lentils, cheese, vegetable extract and mixed herbs into a bowl. Heat the oil in a non stick pan and gently fry the onions and garlic. Mix with the lentils and spoon into a large lightly greased ovenproof dish. Add the water and cover the dish with foil. Cook in the oven at 180°C (350°F) mark 4 for 1 1/2 hours.

261 Kcal/1085 KJ • 16.7 g Protein • 24.1 g Carbohydrate, of which: 4.8 g sugars • 11.5 g Fat, of which: 5.8 g saturates • 0.3 g Sodium • 5.4 g Dietary Fibre

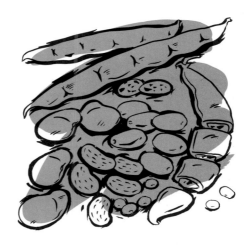

LENTIL BOBOTIE

SERVES 4

10 ml (2 tsp) sunflower oil
2 medium onions, peeled and chopped
1 clove garlic, crushed
15 ml (1 tbsp) curry powder
50 g (2 oz) sultanas
5 ml (1 tsp) dried mixed herbs
250 g (8 oz) red lentils
300 ml ($\frac{1}{2}$ pint) skimmed milk
15 ml (1 tbsp) vinegar
ground black pepper
pinch salt

Heat the oil in a pan and gently fry the onions for 8 minutes. Add the garlic and fry for a further 2 minutes. Mix all the ingredients together in a bowl. Place the mixture in a large greased ovenproof dish and cover with foil. Cook in the oven at 180°C (350°F) mark 4 for 1^3/$_4$ hours.

289 Kcal/1210 KJ • 18.4 g Protein • 49.7 g Carbohydrate, of which: 18.0 g sugars • 3.2 g Fat, of which: 0.4 g saturates • trace Sodium • 9.3 g Dietary Fibre

HUMMUS

SERVES 4

250 g (8 oz) chick peas, cooked
75 ml (5 tbsp) lemon juice
30 ml (2 tbsp) tahini
1 – 2 cloves garlic, crushed
salt
pinch ground cumin

Purée the chick peas, lemon juice, tahini and garlic in a food processor until soft. Season and add water, if necessary.

225 Kcal/940 KJ • 13.4 g Protein • 32.1 g Carbohydrate, of which: 2.7 g sugars • 6.0 g Fat, of which: no saturates • trace Sodium • 13.5 g Dietary Fibre

BLACK BEAN SOUP

SERVES 4

175 g (6 oz) black beans, soaked
10 ml (2 tsp) sunflower oil
1 large onion, peeled and chopped
4 sticks celery, chopped
2 carrots, peeled and chopped
1 clove garlic, crushed
5 ml (1 tsp) ground cumin
ground black pepper
pinch chilli powder (optional)
1.5 litres (2^1/$_2$ pints) vegetable stock

Soak the beans overnight in water. Alternatively place the beans in a large pan, cover with water and bring to the boil cook for 2 minutes, then turn off the heat and leave for 1 hour. Heat in oil in a large saucepan and sauté the onion, celery and carrots for 8 minutes. Add the garlic and spices and cook for a further 2 minutes. Drain the beans, add to the pan with the stock and simmer for 2 hours or until the beans are cooked. Alternatively, the soup can be cooked in a pressure cooker for 45 minutes. Purée the soup in a blender.

179 Kcal/748 KJ • 10.3 g Protein • 27.1 g Carbohydrate, of which: 5.3 g sugars • 3.2 g Fat, of which: 0.3 g saturates • 0.2 g Sodium • 4.1 g Dietary Fibre

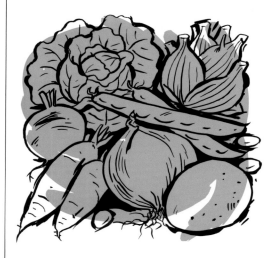

PORK AND BEAN OR COURGETTE AND BEAN GOULASH

SERVES 4

350 g (12 oz) pork fillet, trimmed of fat
15 ml (1 tbsp) soya oil
2 large onions, peeled and chopped
1 green pepper, deseeded and chopped
1 clove garlic, crushed
15 ml (1 tbsp) paprika
sprig of thyme
400 g (14 oz) can chopped tomatoes
15 ml (1 tbsp) tomato purée
400 g (14 oz) cooked kidney beans
75 ml (5 tbsp) water

Cut the pork into medium sized pieces. Heat the oil and brown the meat. Remove from the pan. Gently fry the onions and pepper in the pan for 5 minutes or until soft. Add the garlic and cook for a further minute. Stir in the paprika and thyme and cook for 2 minutes. Return the meat to the pan with the tomatoes, tomato purée, kidney beans and water. Gently simmer for 1 hour.

286 Kcal/1197 KJ • 27.7 g Protein • 25.2 g Carbohydrate, of which: 7.9 g sugars • 9.1 g Fat, of which: 2.7 g saturates • 0.1 g Sodium • 9.6 g Dietary Fibre

Variation: Courgette and bean goulash. For a vegetarian version, use 450 g (1 lb) courgettes instead of the meat, adding them with the garlic.

186 Kcal/777 KJ • 11.4 g Protein • 30.2 g Carbohydrate, of which: 7.8 g sugars • 3.4 g Fat, of which: 0.3 g saturates • trace Sodium • 9.6 g Dietary Fibre

VEGETABLE CHILLI

SERVES 4

15 ml (1 tbsp) olive oil
2 medium onions, peeled and chopped
2 cloves garlic, crushed
225 g (8 oz) carrots, peeled and chopped into chunky sticks
1 large red pepper, deseeded and sliced
100 g (3$\frac{1}{2}$ oz) mushrooms, chopped into chunky pieces
5 ml (1 tsp) ground cumin
5 ml (1 tsp) dried oregano
2.5 ml ($\frac{1}{2}$ tsp) cayenne pepper
10 ml (2 tsp) mild chilli seasoning
225 g (8 oz) can tomatoes
75 g (3 oz) tomato purée
225 g (8 oz) cooked kidney beans
225 g (8 oz) cooked haricot beans
1 bay leaf
300 ml ($\frac{1}{2}$ pint) vegetable stock
ground black pepper

Heat the oil in a large pan and cook the onions until soft, about 5 − 8 minutes. Add the garlic and fry for a further minute. Stir in the vegetables, cover the pan and cook for 2 minutes. Add all the remaining ingredients and simmer for 20 minutes. Remove the bay leaf and serve.

216 Kcal/905 KJ • 12.1 g Protein • 31.2 g Carbohydrate, of which: 11.5 g sugars • 5.7 g Fat, of which: 0.7 g saturates • 0.3 g Sodium • 13.2 g Dietary Fibre

BEAN PATÉ

SERVES 4

15 ml (1 tblsp) sunflower oil
1 onion, peeled and chopped
1 clove garlic, crushed
1.25 ml ($^1/_4$ tsp) ground cumin
1.25 – 2.5 ml ($^1/_4$ – $^1/_2$ tsp) Tabasco sauce
400 g (14 oz) can red kidney beans, drained
100 ml (4 fl oz) water
30 ml (2 tbsp) Greek yogurt
paprika

Heat the oil in a pan and gently cook the onion until well browned, about 10 – 12 minutes. Add the garlic, cumin and Tabasco sauce. Stir in the beans and water, then cook down to a thickened mixture, mashing the beans slightly so that it is fairly smooth. Transfer the pâté to a serving bowl. Spread the yogurt over the top and lightly sprinkle with paprika.

392 Kcal/1638 KJ • 24.0 g Protein • 61.2 g Carbohydrate, of which: 3.7 g sugars • 5.1 g Fat, of which: 0.8 g saturates • trace Sodium • 5.0 g Dietary Fibre

LENTIL AND SPINACH SOUP

SERVES 4

175 g (6 oz) green lentils
10 ml (2 tsp) soya oil
1 large onion, peeled and chopped
5 ml (1 tsp) ground cumin
450 g (1 lb) fresh, thawed or frozen spinach, washed
300 ml ($^1/_2$ pint) vegetable stock
ground black pepper

Cover the lentils with water in a large saucepan. Bring to the boil and simmer for 40 minutes. Heat the oil in a non stick fry pan and cook the onion until just soft, about 5 minutes. Add the cumin and cook for a further 2 minutes. Stir in the spinach and cook until it becomes limp. Drain the lentils and mix with the spinach and stock. Purée the soup in a blender. Reheat, add black pepper to taste and serve.

206 Kcal/862 KJ • 15.4 g Protein • 31.0 g Carbohydrate, of which: 4.0 g sugars • 3.6 g Fat, of which: 0.4 g saturates • 0.3 g Sodium • 5.9 g Dietary Fibre

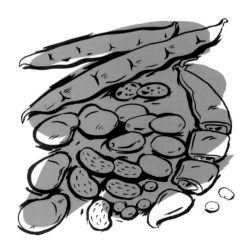

BEAN SALAD (PLUS TUNA OR BACON)

SERVES 4

350 g (12 oz) French beans, trimmed
400 g (14 oz) cooked red kidney beans
225 g (8 oz) cooked chick peas
Dressing:
15 ml (1 tbsp) Greek yogurt
large pinch sugar
ground black pepper
15 ml (1 tbsp) chopped fresh mint (optional)
5 ml (1 tsp) French mustard
15 ml (1 tbls) olive oil
15 ml (1 tbsp) red wine vinegar

Steam the French beans until just tender, about 7 minutes. Put all the beans and chick peas into a large salad bowl. Mix together the dressing ingredients and pour over the beans. Toss to mix together. Allow to stand for 1 hour to let the flavours mix before serving.

157 Kcal/657 KJ • 9.9 g Protein • 21.8 g Carbohydrate, of which: 3.2 g sugars • 4.1 g Fat, of which: 0.6 g saturates • trace Sodium • 11.3 g Dietary Fibre

Variations: Tuna and Bean salad: Add 200 g (7 oz) canned tuna, drained and flaked, to the salad.

217 Kcal/909 KJ • 23.4 g Protein • 21.8 g Carbohydrate, of which: 3.2 g sugars • 4.7 g Fat, of which: 0.6 g saturates • trace Sodium • 11.3 g Dietary Fibre

Bacon and Bean salad: 100 g (4 oz) lean back bacon. Grill. Cut into small pieces and add to the salad.

230 Kcal/962 KJ • 17.5 g Protein • 21.8 g Carbohydrate, of which: 3.2 g sugars • 8.8 g Fat, of which: 2.5 g saturates • 0.6 g Sodium • 11.3 g Dietary Fibre

DHAL

SERVES 4

150 g (5 oz) red lentils
1 cm (1/2 inch) piece unpeeled fresh root ginger, thinly sliced
10 ml (2 tsp) sunflower oil
2 large onions, peeled and finely chopped
2.5 ml (1/2 tsp) ground turmeric
5 ml (1 tsp) ground cumin
5 ml (1 tsp) ground coriander
1.25 ml (1/4 tsp) chilli powder

Place the lentils and ginger in a large saucepan and cover with boiling water. Gently simmer for 30 – 45 minutes until the lentils are soft. Drain and remove the pieces of ginger. Heat the oil in a non stick frying pan and gently cook the onions until soft, about 5 – 8 minutes. Add the spices and cook for a further 2 minutes. Mix the lentils and spices together in a large saucepan and cook over a low heat for 10 minutes, stirring frequently to prevent sticking. Add more water if necessary to prevent sticking. (Dhal should be the consistency of runny porridge).

162 Kcal/675 KJ • 9.9 g Protein • 24.8 g Carbohydrate, of which: 4.8 g sugars • 3.2 g Fat, of which: 0.3 g saturates • trace Sodium • 5.4 g Dietary Fibre

VEGETABLES

MUSHROOMS À LA GRECQUE

SERVES 4

10 ml (2 tsp) olive oil

1 small onion, peeled and finely chopped

1 clove garlic, crushed

150 g (5 oz) tomato purée

300 ml (½ pint) water

1 bay leaf

60 ml (4 tbsp) chopped fresh parsley

10 coriander seeds, tied inside a muslin bag or coffee filter bag to make a bouquet garni

ground black pepper

750 g (1½ lb) mushrooms, thickly sliced

Heat the oil in a pan and gently fry the onion until soft, about 5 minutes. Add the garlic and cook for a further minute. Add the remaining ingredients, except the mushrooms, and simmer for 30 minutes. Add the mushrooms and a little water if necessary, then cook for a further 15 minutes. Remove the bouquet garni before serving.

> 76 Kcal/316 KJ • 4.6 g Protein • 5.4 g Carbohydrate, of which: 5.0 g sugars • 4.1 g Fat, of which: 0.6 g saturates • trace Sodium • 3.0 g Dietary Fibre

STIR FRY VEGETABLES (WITH CHICKEN OR PORK)

SERVES 4

10 ml (2 tsp) sunflower oil

1 large onion, peeled and chopped

2 carrots, peeled and cut into fine matchsticks

2.5 cm (1 inch) piece fresh root ginger, peeled and finely chopped

1 clove garlic, crushed

275 g (10 oz) chicken breast or pork fillet, cut into fine strips (optional)

¼ white cabbage, finely chopped

100 g (3½ oz) mushrooms, sliced

250 g (8 oz) beansprouts

15 ml (1 tbsp) dry sherry

30 ml (2 tbsp) soy sauce

Heat the oil in a wok or large non stick fry pan and stir fry the onion, carrots and ginger for 3 minutes, stirring continuously. Add the garlic and stir for another minute. If using chicken or pork, remove the vegetables from the pan and fry the meat for 3 minutes. Return the vegetables to the pan with the cabbage, mushrooms and beansprouts, and stir-fry for 2 minutes. Add the sherry and soy sauce, then cover and cook for 4 minutes.

> VEGETABLES ONLY
> 71 Kcal/297 KJ • 4.1 g Protein • 7.4 g Carbohydrate, of which: 2.3 g sugars • 2.8 g Fat, of which: 0.4 g saturates • trace Sodium • 2.3 g Dietary Fibre

> WITH CHICKEN OR PORK
> 155 Kcal/645 KJ • 18.2 g Protein • 7.4 g Carbohydrate, of which: 2.3 g sugars • 5.8 g Fat, of which: 1.3 g saturates • trace Sodium • 2.3 g Dietary Fibre

MANGE TOUT AND CARROTS WITH SOY SAUCE

SERVES 4

300 g (10 oz) baby carrots
350 g (12 oz) mangetout trimmed
30 ml (2 tbsp) soy sauce
½ clove garlic, crushed (optional)
1 cm (½ inch) piece fresh root ginger, peeled and chopped (optional)
25 g (1 oz) sunflower seeds, toasted

Remove the tops from the carrots, then scrub them. Bring a large steamer to the boil and steam the carrots for 5 minutes. Add the mange tout and steam for a further 2 minutes. Place the vegetables, soy sauce, garlic and ginger in a large pan and stir for 1 minute until thoroughly mixed. Put into a large bowl and sprinkle with the sunflower seeds.

97 Kcal/404 KJ • 7.3 g Protein • 10.0 g Carbohydrate, of which: 4.7 g sugars • 3.4 g Fat, of which: 0.1 g saturates • 0.2 g Sodium • 14.1 g Dietary Fibre

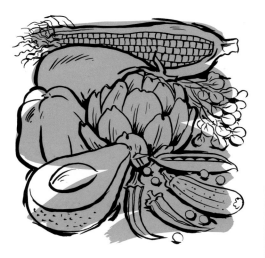

STUFFED PEPPERS

SERVES 4

4 large green peppers, cut in half and deseeded
10 ml (2 tsp) olive oil
2 onions, peeled and chopped
2 cloves garlic, crushed
45 ml (3 tbsp) tomato purée
60 ml (4 tbsp) red wine
75 g (3 oz) cashew nuts
400 g (14 oz) can tomatoes
15 ml (2 tbsp) chopped fresh parsley
15 ml (1 tbsp) chopped fresh thyme
ground black pepper
225 g (8 oz) cooked long grain brown rice

Bring a large pan of water to the boil, then parboil the peppers for 5 minutes. Drain and cool quickly. Put into a large greased ovenproof dish. Heat the oil in a large non stick pan and fry the onions for 8 minutes or until soft. Add the garlic and cook for a further 2 minutes. Add the remaining ingredients, except the rice, and simmer for 20 minutes. Add the rice and thoroughly mix. Stuff the peppers with the mixture. Place any extra mixture around the peppers. Cook in the oven at 180°C (350°F) mark 4 for 25 minutes.

288 Kcal/1212 KJ • 8.9 g Protein • 36.2 g Carbohydrate, of which: 10.8 g sugars • 12.5 g Fat, of which: 0.4 g saturates • trace Sodium • 4.2 g Dietary Fibre

VEGETABLE CURRY

SERVES 4

15 ml (3 tsp) sunflower oil
1 large onion, peeled and chopped
2 celery sticks, chopped
2 cloves garlic, crushed
4 cloves
4 whole green cardamoms
5 ml (1 tsp) ground cumin
2.5 ml ($\frac{1}{2}$ tsp) ground coriander
2.5 ml ($\frac{1}{2}$ tsp) ground turmeric
5 ml (1 tsp) paprika
pinch chilli powder
5 ml (1 tsp) garam marsala
1 parsnip, peeled and chopped
450 g (1 lb) potatoes, scrubbed and chopped
1 courgette, sliced
$\frac{1}{2}$ small cauliflower, broken into florets
100 g ($3\frac{1}{2}$ oz) frozen peas
400 g (14 oz) can chopped tomatoes
ground black pepper
60 ml (4 tbsp) water

Heat 5 ml (1 tsp) oil in a large flame proof casserole and cook the onion and celery over a low heat for 10 minutes. Add the garlic and cloves and cook for a further 2 minutes. Add the remaining oil and spices and cook for 2 minutes. Mix in the vegetables, black pepper and water, and cook gently over a low heat for 35 – 40 minutes until tender.

205 Kcal/855 KJ • 6.9 g Protein • 36.6 g Carbohydrate, of which: 7.1 g sugars • 4.7 g Fat, of which: 0.5 g saturates • trace Sodium • 7.8 g Dietary Fibre

GRILLED SUMMER VEGETABLES

SERVES 4

2 small aubergines
3 courgettes
1 yellow pepper, deseeded
1 red pepper, deseeded
15 ml (1 tbsp) olive oil
15 ml (1 tbsp) wine vinegar
1 clove garlic, crushed
5 ml (1 tsp) chopped fresh oregano
ground black pepper

Cut the aubergine into 0.5 ($\frac{1}{4}$ inch) slices. Cut the courgettes diagonally into 1 cm ($\frac{1}{2}$ inch) slices. Cut the peppers into large slices. Mix the oil, vinegar, garlic, oregano and black pepper in a large bowl. Add the vegetables, cover with the mixture and leave to marinate for at least 1 hour. Cook the vegetables on a barbecue or under a hot grill until just tender, basting frequently.

95 Kcal/398 KJ • 3.5 g Protein • 11.7 g Carbohydrate, of which: 7.0 g sugars • 4.5 g Fat, of which: 0.6 g saturates • trace sodium • 5.2 g Dietary Fibre

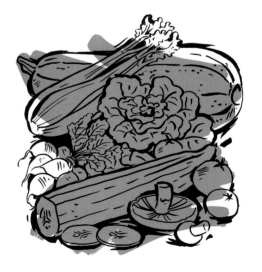

SPINACH AND CHEESE SQUARES

SERVES 4

2 large eggs, size 1 or 2
100 g (3¹/₂ oz) wholemeal flour
275 g (10 oz) frozen chopped spinach, thawed and drained well
450 g (1 lb) cottage cheese
175 g (6 oz) reduced fat Cheddar cheese
ground black pepper

Beat the eggs and wholemeal flour together in a large bowl. Add the spinach, cottage cheese, Cheddar cheese and black pepper. Spoon the mixture into a well greased large ovenproof dish. Bake in the oven at 180°C (350°F) mark 4 for about 45 minutes. Leave to cool for at least 5 minutes before serving.

329 Kcal/1385 KJ • 36.2 g Protein • 22.2 g Carbohydrate, of which: 4.2 g sugars • 11.5 g Fat, of which: 5.5 g saturates • 0.8 g Sodium • 2.2 g Dietary Fibre

GREEN BEANS WITH ALMONDS

SERVES 4

450 g (1 lb) French green beans, topped and tailed
5 ml (1 tsp) sunflower oil
25 g (1 oz) flaked almonds

Bring a large pan of water to the boil. Parboil the beans for 3 minutes, then drain and cool. Heat the oil in a wok or large non stick fry pan and stir the beans for 4 minutes. Add the almonds and stir for a further 3 minutes.

54 Kcal/227 KJ • 2.0 g Protein • 1.5 g Carbohydrate, of which: 1.2 g sugars • 5.0 g Fat, of which: 0.4 g saturates • trace Sodium • 4.5 g Dietary Fibre

VEGETABLE AND FISH KEBABS

SERVES 4

1 red pepper, deseeded and cut into chunks
1 green pepper, deseeded and cut into chunks
3 small courgettes, cut into 2.5 cm (1 inch) chunks
225 g (8 oz) cherry tomatoes
150 (5 oz) button mushrooms
450 g (1 lb) fish, such as monkfish, red mullet, plaice, scallops, baby squid, large raw prawns and langoustine
30 ml (2 tbsp) olive oil
30 ml (2 tbsp) lemon juice
30 ml (2 tbsp) chopped fresh basil
ground black pepper

For best results, partially cook the peppers and courgettes first by blanching in boiling water for a couple of minutes. Drain and cool. Cut the fish into bite-sized pieces. Thread all the vegetables and fish on to skewers, alternating them. Mix the oil, lemon juice, basil and black pepper together. Heat the grill or barbecue. When hot, cook the kebabs for about 10 minutes, basting liberally with the oil mixture.

207 Kcal/867 KJ • 24.6 g Protein • 7.7 g Carbohydrate, of which: 2.5 g sugars • 7.3 g Fat, of which: 1.0 g saturates • 0.2 g Sodium • 2.1 g Dietary Fibre

PEPPER AND POTATO TORTILLA

SERVES 1

2 eggs
10 ml (2 tsp) water
ground black pepper
10 g (⅓ oz) sunflower margarine
75 g (3 oz) cooked potato, sliced
50 g (2 oz) red pepper, chopped

Break the eggs into a bowl, add the water and black pepper and beat lightly. Heat the margarine in a 15 cm (6 inch) omelette pan until slightly smoking, Add the eggs and proceed as for an ordinary omelette. Preheat the grill. While the omelette is still slightly moist, cover the top with the potato and red pepper. Place the omelette under the grill and brown.

320 Kcal/1329 KJ • 17.0 g Protein • 15.9 g Carbohydrate, of which: 1.4 g sugars • 21.4 g Fat, of which: 5.7 g saturates • 0.3 g Sodium • 1.2 g Dietary Fibre

ITALIAN CABBAGE

SERVES 4

1 head white cabbage, chopped
2.5 ml (½ tsp) grated nutmeg

Bring a large saucepan of water to the boil. Add the cabbage and cook for 3 – 4 minutes. Drain and sprinkle with the nutmeg before serving.

45 Kcal/190 KJ • 4.8 g Protein • 6.8 g Carbohydrate, of which: 6.2 g sugars • 0.2 g Fat, of which: no saturates • trace Sodium • 7.9 g Dietary Fibre

POPPY SEED LEEKS

SERVES 4

4 large leeks, washed and sliced
5 ml (1 tsp) sunflower oil
15 ml (1 tbsp) poppy seeds
ground black pepper

Steam the leeks for 3 minutes. Drain. Heat the oil in a wok and cook the poppy seeds for 30 seconds. Add the leeks and black pepper and cook for a further 2 minutes, stirring constantly.

42 Kcal/175 KJ • 2.2 g Protein • 5.4 g Carbohydrate, of which: 5.2 g sugars • 1.5 g Fat, of which: 0.2 g saturates • trace Sodium • 4.4 g Dietary Fibre

GREEN BEANS IN TOMATO SAUCE

SERVES 4

450 g (1 lb) runner beans
15 ml (1 tbsp) olive oil
1 medium onion, peeled and chopped
2 cloves garlic, crushed
200 g (7 oz) canned tomatoes
150 ml (1 tbsp) tomato purée
100 ml (4 fl oz) water
large handful parsley, chopped
large pinch sugar
ground black pepper

Top and tail the beans and remove any strings, if necessary. Cut into 5 cm (2 inch) pieces. Heat the oil in a pan and gently cook the onion until soft, about 5 minutes. Add the garlic and cook for a further 2 minutes. Stir in the tomatoes, tomato purée, water, parsley, sugar and black pepper then cover and simmer for 25 minutes. Add the green beans and cook for a further 15 – 20 minutes until the beans are tender. Serve hot or cold as a starter.

64 Kcal/268 KJ • 2.0 g Protein • 6.1 g Carbohydrate, of which: 5.4 g sugars • 3.8 g Fat, of which: 0.5 g saturates • trace Sodium • 4.8 g Dietary Fibre

AUBERGINE PATÉ

SERVES 4

2 medium aubergines
2 cloves garlic, crushed
15 ml (1 tbsp) oil
30 ml (2 tbsp) pomegranate juice or orange juice
2.5 ml ($\frac{1}{2}$ tsp) paprika
pinch chilli seasoning

Prick the aubergines with a fork and place on a baking tray. Bake in the oven at 180°C (350°F) mark 4 for 30 minutes or until tender. When the aubergines are cooked, remove the skin while hot. Purée the flesh in a food processor with the garlic, oil, pomegranate juice, paprika and chilli. Leave to cool, then serve with pitta bread.

66 Kcal/278 KJ • 1.4 g Protein • 7.1 g Carbohydrate, of which: 6.0 g sugars • 3.9 g Fat, of which: 0.5 g saturates • trace Sodium • 4.4 g Dietary Fibre

SPINACH AND LENTIL OR CHICKEN DHANSAK

SERVES 4

10 ml (2 tsp) sunflower oil
1 large onion, peeled and chopped
2 cloves garlic, crushed
1 green chilli, deseeded and finely chopped
7.5 ml (1$\frac{1}{2}$ tsp) ground cumin
5 ml (1 tsp) ground coriander
5 ml (1 tsp) garam masala
4 cardamoms, crushed
5 ml (1 tsp) ground turmeric
pinch chilli powder
100 g (3$\frac{1}{2}$ oz) red lentils
5 tomatoes, skinned and chopped
300 ml ($\frac{1}{2}$ pint) water
450 g (1 lb) fresh spinach, washed, or frozen spinach
large handful coriander, chopped
small handful mint, chopped
ground black pepper

Heat the oil in a large flameproof casserole and gently cook the onion for 10 minutes or until brown. Add the garlic, chilli and spices, and cook for a further 2 minutes. Stir in the lentils, tomatoes and water, and simmer for 30 minutes, stirring occasionally to prevent the mixture from sticking. Add the spinach, coriander, mint and black pepper and simmer for a further 10 minutes.

167 Kcal/699 KJ • 11.4 g Protein • 24.7 g Carbohydrate, of which: 5.5 g sugars • 3.7 g Fat, of which: 0.3 g saturates • 0.1 g Sodium • 4.8 g Dietary Fibre

Variation: Chicken Dhansak. Add 1 small chicken breast per person. Brown the chicken breasts and add at the same time as the lentils.

283 Kcal/1184 KJ • 33.2 g Protein • 24.7 g Carbohydrate, of which: 5.5 g sugars • 6.9 g Fat, of which: 1.4 g saturates • 0.2 g Sodium • 4.8 g Dietary Fibre

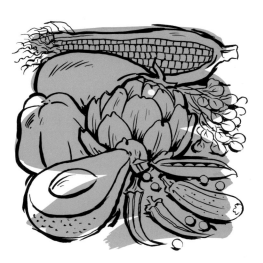

TOMATO AND COURGETTE SOUP

SERVES 4

10 ml (2 tsp) sunflower oil
1 large onion, peeled and chopped
2 cloves garlic, crushed
400 g (14 oz) can tomatoes
450 g (1 lb) courgettes
450 ml (^{3}/$_4$ pint) water
30 ml (2 tbsp) tomato purée
5 ml (1 tsp) sugar
large handful basil, chopped
15 ml (1 tbsp) wine vinegar
ground black pepper

Heat the oil in a large saucepan and cook the onion and garlic until soft, stirring frequently, about 5 – 8 minutes. Add the tomatoes, courgettes, water, tomato purée, sugar, basil, vinegar and black pepper. Simmer for 20 – 25 minutes until all the vegetables are tender. Purée the soup in a blender and serve.

88 Kcal/366 KJ • 4.1 g Protein • 12.5 g Carbohydrate, of which: 7.0 g sugars • 3.0 g Fat, of which: 0.3 g saturates • trace Sodium • 1.8 g Dietary Fibre

CHICKEN WITH WATERCRESS SAUCE

SERVES 4

10 ml (2 tsp) sunflower oil
4 small chicken breasts
2 medium onions, peeled and chopped
100 g (3^1/$_2$ oz) watercress
75 g (3 oz) frozen peas
175 g (6 oz) peeled old potatoes
450 ml (^{3}/$_4$ pint) vegetable or chicken stock
ground black pepper

Heat the oil in a large non stick pan and brown the chicken. Remove the chicken. Add the onions and cook for 5 minutes until just soft. Add the watercress and cook for a further 2 minutes. Return the chicken to the pan and add all the remaining ingredients. Cover and cook for 30 minutes. Remove the chicken and keep warm. Purée the sauce in a blender, then pour over the chicken.

213 Kcal/891 KJ • 24.6 g Protein • 13.8 g Carbohydrate, of which: 4.3 g sugars • 6.9 g Fat, of which: 1.8 g saturates • 0.3 g Sodium • 3.7 g Dietary Fibre

SALAD CRUNCH

ITALIAN SALAD

SERVES 4

6 sticks celery, with green leaves removed
100 g (3½ oz) mushrooms, sliced
1 red pepper, deseeded and chopped
large handful parsley, chopped
juice of 1 lemon

Chop the celery and mix together with the other ingredients in a salad bowl.

14 Kcal/60 KJ • 1.3 g Protein • 1.7 g Carbohydrate, of which: 1.7 g sugars • 0.3 g Fat, of which: 0.1 g saturates • trace Sodium • 2.3 g Dietary Fibre

FENNEL, APRICOT AND WALNUT SALAD

SERVES 4

1 bulb fennel, with green leaves removed
50 g (2 oz) dried no-soak apricots
25 g (1 oz) walnuts

Chop the fennel, apricots and walnuts. Mix together in a salad bowl.

60 Kcal/250 KJ • 1.8 g Protein • 6.5 g Carbohydrate, of which: 6.3 g sugars • 3.2 g Fat, of which: 0.4 g saturates • trace Sodium • 4.4 g Dietary Fibre

MUSHROOM SALAD

SERVES 4

350 g (12 oz) mushrooms, sliced
2 large handfuls chives, chopped
100 g (3½ oz) low fat natural yogurt
10 ml (2 tsp) lemon juice
ground black pepper

Mix the mushrooms, chives, yogurt, lemon juice and black pepper together in a salad bowl. Leave for 1 hour before serving.

26 Kcal/107 KJ • 2.9 g Protein • 1.9 g Carbohydrate, of which: 1.9 g sugars • 0.7 g Fat, of which: 0.2 g saturates • trace Sodium • 2.2 g Dietary Fibre

TURKISH SALAD

SERVES 4

6 tomatoes, cut into small dice
1 cucumber, cut into small dice
1 small mild onion, peeled and finely sliced
large handful mint, chopped
juice of 1 lemon
sprinkling of sumac (optional)

Place the tomatoes, cucumber, onion and mint in a salad bowl. Squeeze the lemon juice over them and mix with the salad. Sprinkle with the sumac to give colour.

22 Kcal/94 KJ • 1.3 g Protein • 4.3 g Carbohydrate, of which: 4.3 g sugars • 0.1 g Fat, of which: trace saturates • trace Sodium • 1.6 g Dietary Fibre

WATERCRESS AND ORANGE SALAD

SERVES 4

100 g (3½ oz) watercress, washed
2 large oranges

Break up the watercress and place in a large salad bowl. Cut off both ends of each orange with a sharp knife. With a small knife, carefully cut off the skin and pith. Cut into thin slices with a bread knife and cut each slice into quarters. Mix the orange pieces with the watercress and serve.

26 Kcal/110 KJ • 1.2 g Protein • 5.7 g Carbohydrate, of which: 5.6 g sugars • no Fat, of which: no saturates • trace Sodium • 2.1 g Dietary Fibre

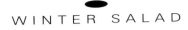

WINTER SALAD

SERVES 4

½ red cabbage, finely sliced
1 small onion, peeled and finely sliced
1 green pepper, deseeded and finely sliced
1 red pepper, deseeded and finely sliced
45 ml (3 tbsp) French dressing (see page 144)

Mix all the ingredients together in a large bowl.

107 Kcal/444 KJ • 2.4 g Protein • 5.7 g Carbohydrate, of which: 5.7 g sugars • 8.5 g Fat, of which: 1.2 g saturates • 0.1 Sodium • 4.2 g Dietary Fibre

CARROT AND NUT SALAD

SERVES 4

450 g (1 lb) carrots, peeled
75 g (3 oz) natural roasted peanuts, unsalted
2 large handfuls parsley, chopped
30 ml (2 tbsp) freshly squeezed orange juice
30 ml (2 tbsp) French dressing (see page 144)
ground black pepper
10 ml (2 tsp) orange flower water (optional)

Grate the carrots. Finely chop the nuts. Mix the nuts with the carrots, parsley, orange juice, dressing, black pepper and orange flower water in a large salad bowl.

185 Kcal/770 KJ • 5.4 g Protein • 8.4 g Carbohydrate, of which: 7.4 g sugars • 14.7 g Fat, of which: 2.5 g saturates • 0.2 Sodium • 4.8 g Dietary Fibre

GARDEN SALAD

SERVES 4

2 handfuls Quattro Stagioni
2 large handfuls red oak leaf lettuce
2 large handfuls Cos lettuce
handful Greek cress
handful rocket
handful coriander leaves
handful parsley leaves

Clean and wash all the salad. Remove and discard any bruised or yellowed leaves, then dry thoroughly. Place in a salad large bowl and serve.

8 Kcal/31 KJ • 0.6 g Protein • 0.8 g Carbohydrate, of which: 0.8 g sugars • 0.3 g Fat, of which: no saturates • trace Sodium • 0.9 g Dietary Fibre

LEMON COLESLAW

SERVES 4

½ white cabbage
75 g (3 oz) sultanas or raisins
juice of 1 lemon

Finely chop the cabbage and place in a large salad bowl with the sultanas. Squeeze over the lemon juice and mix with the cabbage and sultanas.

65 Kcal/275 KJ • 1.9 g Protein • 15.3 g Carbohydrate, of which: 15.3 g sugars • no Fat, of which: no saturates • trace Sodium • 3.3 g Dietary Fibre

INSALATA DI MARE – SEAFOOD SALAD

SERVES 4

225 g (8 oz) fresh or frozen squid, prepared and cut into rings
100 g (3½ oz) peeled prawns
225 g (8 oz) unpeeled prawns
large handful parsley, chopped
few leaves basil, chopped
juice of 1 lemon
15 ml (1 tbsp) olive oil
ground black pepper
1 green lettuce
1 red lollo rosso lettuce
2 red peppers, deseeded and sliced
4 tomatoes, sliced

Place the seafood in a large salad bowl. Mix together the parsley, basil, lemon juice, oil and black pepper. Pour over the fish, stir and leave for at least 1 hour in the fridge for the flavours to mix. Remove and discard any bruised or yellowed leaves from the lettuces. Wash and thoroughly dry them. Once the fish has marinated, tear the lettuce into shreds and add to the bowl with the red peppers and tomatoes. Toss, bringing the unpeeled prawns to the surface.

143 Kcal/600 KJ • 19.6 g Protein • 4.2 g Carbohydrate, of which: 4.2 g sugars • 5.4 g Fat, of which: 0.6 g saturates • 0.8 g Sodium • 2.3 g Dietary Fibre

SPINACH AND HAM OR EGG SALAD

SERVES 4

450 g (1 lb) spinach
150 g (5 oz) lean thick-cut honey roast ham
45 ml (3 tbsp) French dressing (see page 144)

Remove and discard the tough spinach stalks and any bruised or yellowed leaves. Tear the large leaves in half or into thirds. Wash the spinach in at least two changes of water and spin dry. Place the spinach in a large salad bowl. Cut the ham into small bite sized pieces. Gently heat the French dressing until just warm, pour over the spinach and toss quickly. Mix in the ham.

148 Kcal/615 KJ • 10.5 g Protein • 4.2 g Carbohydrate, of which: trace sugars • 10.5 g Fat, of which: • 1.8 g saturates • 0.7 Sodium • trace Dietary Fibre

Variation: Instead of the ham add 2 hard boiled eggs, finely diced.

148 Kcal/614 KJ • 7.4 g Protein • 4.2 g Carbohydrate, of which: trace sugars • 11.9 g Fat, of which: 2.1 g saturates • 0.2 g Sodium • trace Dietary Fibre

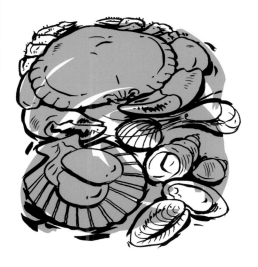

THAI CHICKEN SALAD

SERVES 4

2 lettuce
4 small roasted chicken breasts
4 large tomatoes, cut into eighths
1 yellow pepper, deseeded and sliced
6 spring onions, finely sliced
100 g (3½ oz) beansprouts
Dressing:
15 ml (1 tbsp) tahini
15 ml (1 tbsp) sunflower oil
15 ml (1 tbsp) white vinegar
5 ml (1 tsp) sugar
pinch chilli powder

Remove and discard any lettuce leaves that are bruised or yellowed. Wash and thoroughly dry the lettuce, then place in a large salad bowl. Chop the chicken into bite sized pieces and mix with the tomatoes, pepper, spring onions and beansprouts. Add to the bowl. Mix together the dressing ingredients. Pour over the salad, toss and serve.

237 Kcal/991 KJ • 29 g Protein • 6.4 g Carbohydrate, of which: 4.9 g sugars • 11.0 g Fat, of which: 2.3 g saturates • trace Sodium • 2.1 g Dietary Fibre

SALAD NIÇOISE

SERVES 4

1 – 2 lettuces, depending on size
4 large ripe tomatoes, sliced
225 g (8 oz) French beans, cooked
45 ml (3 tbsp) French dressing (see page 144)
200 g (7 oz) canned tuna in brine, drained
50 g (2 oz) canned anchovies in oil, drained
2 eggs, hard boiled and halved
12 black olives

Remove and discard any lettuce leaves that are bruised or yellowed. Wash and thoroughly dry the lettuce, then place in a large salad bowl. Add the tomatoes, beans and French dressing, then gently mix together. Arrange the remaining ingredients over the top of the salad.

294 Kcal/221 KJ • 17.0 g Protein • 3.3 g Carbohydrate, of which: 3.2 g sugars • 23.8 g Fat, of which: 4.2 g saturates • 0.6 g Sodium • 4.1 g Dietary Fibre

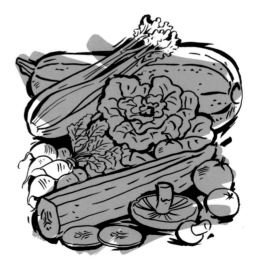

AVOCADO, PRAWN OR WALNUT, APPLE AND CELERY SALAD

SERVES 4

2 lettuce
1 avocado, stoned, peeled and diced
350 g (12 oz) peeled prawns
1 apple, cored and diced
$^1/_2$ bunch of celery, chopped
30 ml (2 tbsp) French dressing (see page 144)
ground black pepper
juice of 1 lemon

Remove and discard any lettuce leaves that are bruised or yellowed. Wash and thoroughly dry the lettuce, then place in a large salad bowl. Place all the ingredients in the bowl, squeezing over the lemon juice, and toss.

247 Kcal/1030 KJ • 22.3 g Protein • 4.7 g Carbohydrate, of which: 4.7 g sugars • 15.7 g Fat, of which: 1.9 g saturates • 1.5 g Sodium • 2.6 g Dietary Fibre

Variation: Instead of the prawns use 50 g (2 oz) chopped walnuts in the salad.

232 Kcal/963 KJ • 4.1 g Protein • 5.4 g Carbohydrate, of which: 5.1 g sugars • 21.8 g Fat, of which: 2.6 g saturates • 0.1 Sodium • 3.3 g Dietary Fibre

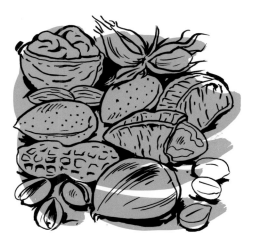

DESSERTS

RASPBERRY SORBET

SERVES 4

450 g (1 lb) fresh raspberries or frozen raspberries, thawed

100 g (3½ oz) caster sugar

150 ml (¼ pint) water

Juice of 1 lemon

1 egg white (optional)

Purée the raspberries and sieve, if preferred. Put the sugar and water in a saucepan and stir over a gentle heat until the sugar has dissolved. Turn up the heat and boil fast for 5 minutes until a sticky syrup forms. When the syrup has cooled, mix it with the fruit purée and lemon juice. Freeze in an ice cream maker for 20 minutes. Alternatively, place the mixture in a bowl in the freezer until beginning to freeze around the edges. Whisk the egg white and fold into the part frozen mixture. Return the sorbet to the freezer until frozen. Variations. Use other fruit, such as strawberries, blackcurrants, redcurrants, blackberries, gooseberries or kiwi fruit. Alternatively, use the flesh of 2 large ripe mangos, or 450 g (1 lb) rhubarb or 450 g (1 lb) apricots.

128 Kcal/538 KJ • 1.1 g Protein • 33.0 g Carbohydrate, of which: 33.0 g sugars • no Fat, of which: no saturates • trace Sodium • 8.3 g Dietary Fibre

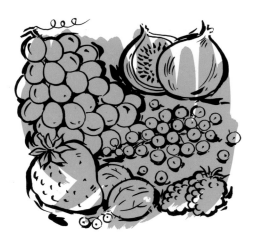

ALMOND BISCUITS

MAKES ABOUT 20

These little biscuits will keep for a couple of weeks in an airtight tin, so there is no need to eat them all at once. Alternatively, freeze them for up to 2 months.

150 g (5 oz) ground almonds

150 g (5 oz) caster sugar

25 g (1 oz) plain flour

generous 30 ml (2 tbsp) egg white

Place all the ingredients in a large bowl. Mix together, then knead the paste. If the mixture still seems dry, add a little more egg white. Roll small balls of paste between floured hands. When smooth, place on a greased baking tray and flatten with the back of a fork. Bake in the oven at 180°C (350°F) mark 4 for 10 – 15 minutes or until just browned underneath.

129 Kcal/544 KJ • 3.1 g Protein • 23.9 g Carbohydrate, of which: 5.8 g sugars • 3.0 g Fat, of which: 0.2 g saturates • trace Sodium • 1.8 g Dietary Fibre

STRAWBERRY YOGURT ICE CREAM

SERVES 4

225 g (8 oz) strawberries

75 g (3 oz) sugar

450 g (16 oz) low fat natural yogurt

1 egg white (optional)

Purée the strawberries and sugar, then sieve if preferred. Mix with the yogurt. Freeze in an ice cream maker for 20 minutes. Alternatively, place the mixture in the freezer until just beginning to freeze around the edges. Whisk the egg white and fold into the part frozen mixture. Return the ice cream to the freezer until frozen.

152 Kcal/636 KJ • 6.0 g Protein • 32.0 g Carbohydrate, of which: 32.0 g sugars • 1.0 g Fat, of which: no saturates • trace Sodium • 1.2 g Dietary Fibre

FRESH FRUIT PLATTER

SERVES 4

Selection of fruit such as:
½ watermelon
2 pears
2 peaches
225 g (8 oz) black seedless grapes
plenty of ice cubes
mint leaves for decoration

Cut the melon into small pieces and remove some of the seeds using a small, sharp knife. Cut the pears and peaches in half and remove the stone or core. Cut each piece into three and further divide each piece in half. Crush the ice in a food processor and turn out onto a large serving plate, leaving any water in the processor. Alternatively, put the ice cubes into a thick plastic bag and crush with a rolling pin. Arrange the fruit on top of the ice and decorate with the mint leaves. Serve by giving each person a fork to spear the fruit of their choice.

102 Kcal/436 KJ • 1.2 g Protein • 25.9 g Carbohydrate, of which: 25.9 g sugars • no Fat, of which: no saturates • trace Sodium • 2.8 g Dietary Fibre

FRUIT PARCELS

SERVES 4

6 apricots
1 apple, preferably Cox's or Braeburn
½ small pineapple
200 ml (7 fl oz) apple and mango juice or orange juice

Cut the apricots in half and remove the stone. Cut the apple in half, remove the core, then cut each piece into six. Remove the outside of the pineapple and the core. Cut into thick slices, then cut each slice into three. Arrange a mixture of the fruit onto 23 cm (9 inch) squares of foil with grease proof paper squares on the inside. Divide the fruit juice between the parcels. Fold the foil to completely enclose the fruit. Bake in the oven at 180°C (350°F) mark 4 for 25 minutes. Variation: For a special occasion, substitute 15 ml (1 tbsp) fruit juice with Calvados or brandy.

86 Kcal/359 KJ • 1.2 g Protein • 21.5 g Carbohydrate, of which: 21.5 g sugars • no Fat, of which: no saturates • 3.2 g Sodium • 2.9 g Dietary Fibre

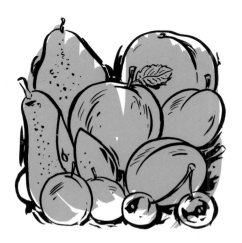

PEACH BRULÉE

SERVES 4

6 large fairly ripe peaches

50 ml (2 fl oz) orange juice

125 g (5 oz) Greek yogurt

75 g (3 oz) low fat natural yogurt

40 – 50 g (1½ – 2 oz) soft brown sugar,
according to size of dish

Remove the skin from the peaches. If the peaches are ripe, simply pull off the skin. Alternatively, skin by cutting a cross in the bottom of each peach and putting into a large bowl of just boiled water. Leave for 4 – 5 minutes, then remove from the bowl and pull off the skin. Cut the peaches in half, then slice and place them in a deep flameproof dish. Pour over the orange juice. Mix together the yogurts. Cover the peaches with the yogurt and sprinkle with the sugar. Heat the grill and place the dish under it. When the sugar has melted and just started to bubble, remove from the grill. Leave to cool. Place in the refrigerator and leave for at least 1 hour. Variation: For a special occasion, spoon 45 ml (3 tbsp) brandy over the peaches before covering with the yogurt.

142 Kcal/598 KJ • 4.5 g Protein • 26.8 g Carbohydrate, of which: 26.8 g sugars • 2.6 g Fat, of which: 1.5 g saturates • trace Sodium • 1.8 g Dietary Fibre

DRIED FRUIT SALAD

SERVES 4

225 g (8 oz) dried, no-soak fruit

1 cinnamon stick

2 cloves

juice of 1 lemon

1 cooking apple, peeled, cored and sliced

50 g (2 oz) raisins

grated nutmeg

Cover the fruit with water in a pan, then add the cinnamon, cloves and lemon juice. Cook for 10 minutes. Add the apple, raisins and nutmeg and cook for a further 5 minutes. Leave for 10 minutes in the pan before serving.

156 Kcal/658 KJ • 2.4 g Protein • 38.9 g Carbohydrate, of which: 38.8 g sugars • no Fat, of which: no saturates • trace Sodium • 12.5 g Dietary Fibre

PEAR WITH FRESH GINGER

SERVES 4

6 large pears, peeled, cored and sliced

2.5 cm (1 inch) piece fresh root ginger, peeled and grated

150 ml (¼ pint) pineapple juice

Place the pear slices in a bowl. Mix the ginger with the pineapple juice, pour over the pears and serve.

87 Kcal/372 KJ • 0.6 g Protein • 22.5 g Carbohydrate, of which: 22.5 g sugars • no Fat, of which: no saturates • trace Sodium • 3.9 g Dietary Fibre

PEACHES STUFFED WITH ALMONDS

SERVES 4

4 large ripe peaches
50 g (2 oz) ground almonds
25 g (1 oz) caster sugar
1 egg white
100 ml (4 fl oz) orange juice

Remove the stone and skin from the peaches (see page 136 under Peach Brûlée). Place the peaches in a single layer in a deep ovenproof dish. Mix together the almonds, sugar and some of the egg white to form a stiff paste. Using a teaspoon, fill the centre of the peaches with the almond mixture. Pour in the orange juice and cover the dish with foil. Cook in the oven at 190°C (375°F) mark 5 for 25 minutes or until the peaches are tender. Remove cover and cook for a further 5 minutes. Variation: For a special occasion, add 5 ml (1 tsp) of cocoa powder to the almond mixture and use some white wine instead of orange juice.

149 Kcal/628 KJ • 3.7 g Protein • 19.7 g Carbohydrate, of which: 19.7 g sugars • 6.7 g Fat, of which: 0.5 g saturates • trace Sodium • 3.0 g Dietary Fibre

SIMPLE TRIFLE

SERVES 4

350 g (12 oz) fatless sponge
225 g (8 oz) frozen strawberries, thawed
1 large banana
45 ml (3 tbsp) orange juice
250 g (9 oz) Greek yogurt
15 g (½ oz) flaked almonds

Cut the sponge into 5 cm (2 inch) squares and place in a medium serving bowl. Place the strawberries on top of the sponge. Peel and slice the banana and place over the strawberries. Pour the orange juice over. Cover the fruit with the yogurt. Sprinkle with flaked almonds and place in the refrigerator for at least 30 minutes before serving.

390 Kcal/1646 KJ • 14.2 g Protein • 57.5 g Carbohydrate, of which: 37.5 g sugars • 13.1 g Fat, of which: 5.2 g saturates • 0.1 g Sodium • 3.4 g Dietary Fibre

BANANA CREAM

SERVES 4

75 g (3 oz) dried no-soak apricots
2 ripe bananas
300 g (10 oz) low fat yogurt

Chop up the apricots and divide between four ramekins. Purée the bananas with the yogurt in a blender. Divide the yogurt mixture between the ramekins. Serve.

111 Kcal/467 KJ • 5.3 g Protein • 22.3 g Carbohydrate, of which: 21.0 g sugars • 0.8 g Fat, of which: 0.4 g saturates • trace Sodium • 6.0 g Dietary Fibre

WALNUT STUFFED PEARS

SERVES 4

4 large ripe pears, peeled, cored and cut in half
50 g (2 oz) sultanas, roughly chopped
50 g (2 oz) walnuts, finely chopped
40 g (1½ oz) soft brown sugar
1 egg white
150 ml (¼ pint) pear or apple juice

Place the pears in a greased deep baking dish. Mix together the sultanas, walnuts, brown sugar, egg white and 15 ml (1 tbsp) fruit juice. Spoon the mixture into the pear cavities. Pour over the remainder of the fruit juice and cover the dish with foil. Bake in the oven at 190°C (375°F) mark 5 for 40 minutes or until tender. Remove the foil and cook for a further 5 minutes.

220 Kcal/929 KJ • 3.0 g Protein • 40.2 g Carbohydrate, of which: 40.0 g sugars • 6.4 g Fat, of which: 0.7 g saturates • trace Sodium • 5.4 g Dietary Fibre

FRUIT KEBABS

SERVES 4

1 banana
1 apple, peeled and cored
½ pineapple
100 g (3½ oz) seedless grapes
10 ml (2 tsp) honey
juice of ½ lemon

Peel the banana and cut into four. Cut the apple into bite sized pieces. Remove the outside of the pineapple, core and cut into bite sized pieces. Place all the fruit in a large bowl. Mix together the honey and lemon juice. Pour over the fruit and mix together. Thread the fruit on to small bamboo skewers. Serve. Variations: Use other fruits such as strawberries, apricots, cherries, melon and kiwi fruit. Alternatively serve hot, heat a grill or barbecue and cook the kebabs for 7 minutes. Turn once or twice during the cooking time.

91 Kcal/382 KJ • 1.0 g Protein • 23.0 g Carbohydrate, of which: 22.3 g sugars • 0.1 g Fat, of which: no saturates • trace Sodium • 2.4 g Dietary Fibre

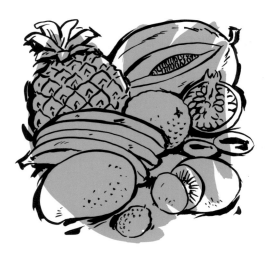

CHEESECAKE

350 g (12 oz) medium fat curd cheese
100 g (3½ oz) granulated sugar
4 eggs, beaten
25 g (1 oz) plain flour
2.5 ml (½ tsp) baking powder
grated rind and juice of 1 lemon
50 g (2 oz) raisins

Grease a deep 15 cm (6 inch) cake tin and line with greaseproof paper. Beat together the cheese and sugar, then gradually add the eggs. Sift the flour and baking powder, and add to the mixture. Stir in the lemon rind, juice and raisins. Pour the mixture into the tin. Bake in the oven at 160°C (325°F) mark 3 for 1 hour or until firm. Serve with a fruit sauce (see page 140).

199 Kcal/832 KJ • 8.3 g Protein • 21.1 g Carbohydrate, of which: 18.7 g sugars • 9.7 g Fat, of which: 4.9 g saturates • trace Sodium • 0.5 g Dietary Fibre

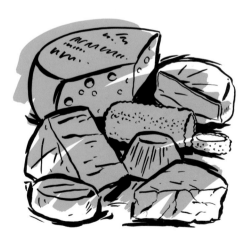

FRUIT SAUCES

Children love dipping pieces of fresh fruit into these sauces. Alternatively, use them instead of cream. For a very special occasion (unless you are trying to lose weight) try the raspberry sauce over chocolate cake! Berry sauces without the yogurt are particularly good served hot.

Nutritional values apply to the whole recipe; not per serving.

MANGO SAUCE

2 mangos
45 ml (3 tbsp) apple or orange juice

Cut the mangos in half and remove the stone with a sharp knife. Peel the mangoes, then place the flesh in a blender with the fruit juice. Purée until smooth.

> *221 Kcal/927 KJ • 2.1 g Protein • 57.0 g Carbohydrate, of which: 57.0 g sugars • no Fat, of which: no saturates • trace Sodium • 4.8 g Dietary Fibre*

RASPBERRY SAUCE

150 g (5 oz) raspberries
30 ml (2 tbsp) Greek yogurt

Purée the rasberries and yogurt in a blender. If you want to remove the pips, push the mixture through a sieve.

> *101 Kcal/420 KJ • 4.9 g Protein • 9.5 g Carbohydrate, of which: 9.5 g sugars • 5.0 g Fat, of which: 2.7 g saturates • trace Sodium • 11.1 g Dietary Fibre*

RHUBARB SAUCE

350 g (12 oz) rhubarb
25 g (1 oz) sugar

Cut the ends off the rhubarb and chop into 2.5 cm (1 inch) pieces. Place the rhubarb pieces in a saucepan and just cover with water. Add the sugar. Bring to the boil and simmer for about 8 minutes or until mushy. Purée in a blender. Variation: make with gooseberries, blackberries, blackcurrants or a mixed fruit sauce of currants and berries.

> *120 Kcal/503 KJ • 2.1 g Protein • 29.8 g Carbohydrate, of which: 29.8 g sugars • no Fat, of which: no saturates • trace Sodium • 9.1 g Dietary Fibre*

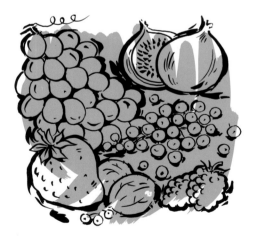

BASICS

Nutritional values apply to the whole recipe; not per serving.

LEMON MARINADE

Suitable for pork, chicken and fish.

15 ml (1 tbsp) sunflower oil
1 clove garlic, crushed
juice of ½ lemon
ground black pepper
30 ml (2 tbsp) chopped fresh herbs or 2.5 ml (½ tsp) dried mixed herbs

Mix all the ingredients together and leave to marinate for at least 30 minutes. Cook over a barbecue, under a grill or in the oven at 200°C (400°F) mark 6. Variation: Try spices instead of the herbs.

142 Kcal/585 KJ • 0.3 g Protein • 1.7 g Carbohydrate, of which: 0.8 g sugars • 15.0 g Fat, of which: 2.0 g saturates • trace Sodium • no Dietary Fibre

YOGURT TANDOORI MARINADE

Suitable for chicken, fish, lamb and beef.

10 ml (2 tsp) sunflower oil
150 ml (5 oz) low fat natural yogurt
5 ml (1 tsp) ground cumin
1.25 ml (¼ tsp) ground turmeric
1.25 ml (¼ tsp) chilli powder
5 ml (1 tsp) ground coriander
5 ml (1 tsp) garam marsala
5 ml (1 tsp) paprika
1 large clove garlic, crushed

Mix all the ingredients together and leave to marinate for at least 1 hour. Cook over a barbecue under a grill or in the oven at 230°C (450°F) mark 8.

229 Kcal/953 KJ • 9.7 g Protein • 18.0 g Carbohydrate, of which: 11.3 g sugars • 13.7 g Fat, of which: 2.0 g saturates • 0.1 g Sodium • no Dietary Fibre

SOY SAUCE MARINADE

Suitable for chicken, pork, lamb and beef.

30 ml (2 tbsp) soy sauce
15 ml (1 tbsp) sunflower oil
1 clove garlic, crushed
5 ml (1 tsp) ground cumin
5 ml (1 tsp) ground coriander
ground black pepper

Mix all the ingredients together and leave to marinate for at least 1 hour. Cook over a barbecue, under a grill or in the oven. Variations: Experiment with other spices.

198 Kcal/818 KJ • 3.3 g Protein • 8.1 g Carbohydrate, of which: no sugars • 17.2 g Fat, of which: 2.1 g saturates • trace Sodium • no Dietary Fibre

DRIED FRUIT AND NUT STUFFING

5 ml (1 tsp) sunflower oil
1 onion, peeled and chopped
2 small cooking apples, peeled and chopped
5 ml (1 tsp) ground cinnamon
50 g (2 oz) dried no-soak prunes, chopped
50 g (2 oz) dried no-soak apricots, chopped
50 g (2 oz) dried no-soak peaches, chopped
50 g (2 oz) raisins
100 g (4 oz) almonds
45 ml (3 tbsp) water

Heat the oil in a non stick pan and fry the onions until soft, about 5 – 8 minutes. Add the apples and cook for 3 minutes. Cover and cook for a further 2 minutes. Add the rest of the ingredients and cook for 5 minutes.

1036 Kcal/4351 KJ • 23.0 g Protein • 112.0 g Carbohydrate, of which: 111.0 g sugars • 59.0 g Fat, of which: 4.9 g saturates • trace Sodium • 43.6 g Dietary Fibre

TOMATO SAUCE

Serve with pasta and hamburgers. Alternatively, add vegetables such as courgettes or aubergines and cook to make a pasta sauce.

10 ml (2 tsp) olive oil
1 medium onion, peeled and chopped
1 clove garlic, crushed
400 g (14 oz) can chopped tomatoes
15 ml (1 tbsp) tomato purée
pinch mixed herbs
pinch sugar
ground black pepper

Heat the oil in a pan and gently brown the onion, over a low heat for about 10 minutes, stirring occasionally. Add the garlic and cook for a further 2 minutes. Stir in the tomatoes, tomato purée, mixed herbs, sugar and black pepper. Cook for 20 minutes or until slightly thickened.

238 Kcal/995 KJ • 7.4 g Protein • 24.3 g Carbohydrate, of which: 24.0 g sugars • 13.0 g Fat, of which: 1.8 g saturates • 0.1 g Sodium • 6.5 g Dietary Fibre

CITRUS SPREAD

1 lemon
100 g (3½ oz) medium fat cream cheese
25 g (1 oz) caster sugar

Finely grate the rind from the lemon and mix with the cheese. Squeeze the juice from the lemon. Add 15 ml (1 tbsp) of the lemon juice and the sugar to the cheese. Keep in the refrigerator.

561 Kcal/2336 KJ • 18.7 g Protein • 60.1 g Carbohydrate, of which: 60.1 g sugars • 29.0 g Fat, of which: 18.2 g saturates • trace Sodium • no Dietary Fibre

RAITA

½ cucumber
150 ml (5 oz) low fat natural yogurt
pinch paprika

Grate the cucumber and leave to drain in a colander. To speed up the process, use a wooden spoon to press out the moisture. Mix the cucumber with the yogurt and place in a bowl. Sprinkle with paprika.

114 Kcal/480 KJ • 9.5 g Protein • 16.7 g Carbohydrate, of which: 16.7 g sugars • 1.5 g Fat, of which: 0.8 g saturates • 0.2 g Sodium • 1.2 g Dietary Fibre

RED PEPPER SAUCE

10 ml (2 tsp) sunflower oil
2 small onions, peeled and chopped
2 red peppers, deseeded and chopped
couple of sprigs thyme, chopped
200 ml (7 fl oz) vegetable stock
ground black pepper

Heat the oil in a pan and gently cook the onions for about 5 minutes until soft. Add the peppers and cook for a further 4 minutes. Stir in the thyme, vegetable stock and black pepper, then cook for 20 minutes. Purée in a blender and serve. Ideal with pasta, grilled pork chops or oven baked chicken.

87 Kcal/360 KJ • 2.0 g Protein • 8.0 g Carbohydrate, of which: 8.0 g sugars • 5.5 g Fat, of which: 0.7 g saturates • trace Sodium • 2.4 g Dietary Fibre

TOMATO SALSA

450 g (1 lb) ripe tomatoes, skinned and deseeded
1 small onion, peeled and finely chopped
1 – 3 green chillies, deseeded and finely chopped
15 ml (1 tbsp) wine vinegar
ground black pepper
pinch sugar
30 ml (2 tbsp) chopped fresh coriander or parsley

Finely chop the tomatoes by hand or put in a food processor but be careful not to overblend. Mix with the remaining ingredients. This will keep for up to a week in the refrigerator. Variation: Use 400 g (14 oz) can chopped tomatoes in the winter (it doesn't make quite such a good salsa.)

182 Kcal/761 KJ • 5.7 g Protein • 18.5 g Carbohydrate, of which: 17.7 g sugars • 10.0 g Fat, of which: 1.4 g saturates • 0.1 g Sodium • 5.2 g Dietary Fibre

MANGO AND TOMATO SALSA

1 mango
225 g (8 oz) ripe tomatoes, skinned and deseeded
1 green chilli, deseeded and finely chopped
15 ml (1 tbsp) chopped fresh mint
15 ml (1 tbsp) chopped fresh coriander
juice of 1 lime
15 ml (1 tbsp) olive oil
pinch sugar
ground black pepper

Cut the mango in half, take out the stone and remove the skin. Finely chop the mango flesh and tomatoes. Mix with the remaining ingredients.

266 Kcal/1114 KJ • 3.2 g Protein • 35.2 g Carbohydrate, of which: 34.0 g sugars • 13.4 g Fat, of which: 1.8 g saturates • trace Sodium • 5.8 g Dietary Fibre

PICA DE GALLO TOMATO RELISH

Anne first tried this in Jackson, Wyoming. It is a great boost to any dish but is particularly good with grilled fish, chicken or beef and warm pitta bread. For those on a diet, it adds flavour without too many calories!

$^1/_2$ sweet onion, peeled and finely chopped
2 tomatoes, finely diced
1 – 3 serrano chillies, deseeded and finely chopped
15 ml (1 tbsp) white vinegar
15 ml (1 tbsp) chopped fresh coriander

Combine all the ingredients together in a bowl. Leave for at least 30 minutes for the flavors to mingle.

37.7 Kcal/158 KJ • 2.1 g Protein • 7.0 g Carbohydrate, of which: 6.3 g sugars • 0.1 g Fat, of which: no saturates • trace Sodium • 2.6 g Dietary Fibre

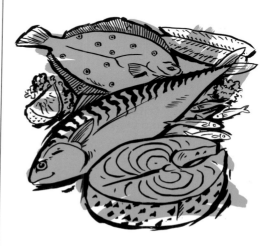

FRENCH DRESSING

30 ml (2 tbsp) olive oil
30 ml (2 tbsp) wine or sherry vinegar
2.5 ml ($\frac{1}{2}$ tsp) French mustard
pinch sugar
salt
ground black pepper

Mix all the ingredients together. Variations: Poppy seed dressing: Add 10 ml (2 tsp) poppy seeds to the dressing. Lemon dressing: Use freshly squeezed lemon juice instead of the vinegar. Soy sauce dressing: Mix together some chopped fresh root ginger, 1 clove crushed garlic, 15 ml (1 tbsp) sunflower or sesame oil, 15 ml (1 tbsp) dry sherry, 15 ml (1 tbsp) soy sauce and a pinch of sugar. Spicy dressing: Add 1 clove crushed garlic and a pinch of chilli powder. Use white vinegar instead of wine vinegar. Mayonnaise dressing: Use 30 ml (2 tbsp) mayonnaise instead of the oil. Herb dressing: Add 30 ml (2 tbsp) chopped fresh herbs, such as basil or mint.

260 Kcal/1089 KJ • 1.0 g Protein • 4.0 g Carbohydrate, of which: 3.3 g sugars • 26.9 g Fat, of which: 3.7 g saturates • trace Sodium • no Dietary Fibre

CAJUN SPICE MIX

Suitable for fish or chicken.

1.25 ml ($\frac{1}{4}$ tsp) chilli powder
15 ml (1 tbsp) paprika
15 ml (1 tbsp) ground cumin
10 ml (2 tsp) ground black pepper
15 ml (1 tbsp) dried oregano

Mix all the ingredients together. Coat fish or meat in the mixture. Cook under the grill or on the barbecue. Lightly brush with oil during cooking.

WEST INDIES MARINADE RUB

Suitable for all meats.

15 ml (1 tbsp) curry powder
15 ml (1 tbsp) ground cumin
1.25 ml ($\frac{1}{4}$ tsp) chilli powder
7.5 ml ($\frac{1}{2}$ tsp) ground black pepper
15 ml (1 tbsp) paprika
2.5 ml ($\frac{1}{2}$ tsp) ground mixed spice

Mix all the ingredients together. Coat meat in the mixture. Cook under the grill or on the barbecue. Lightly brush with oil during cooking.

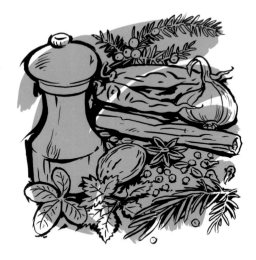

SPECIAL DISHES FOR ENTERTAINING

FISH STEW

15 ml (1 tbsp) olive oil
1 onion, peeled and diced
3 cloves garlic, crushed
8 shallots, peeled
piece of orange rind, blanched (optional)
750 g (1½ lb) ripe tomatoes, skinned and roughly chopped
1 kg (2 lb) prepared fish, such as baby squid, monkfish, prawns, scallops, cod, huss
300 ml (½ pint) fish or vegetable stock
300 ml (½ pint) boiling water
sprig thyme
15 – 30 ml (1 – 2 tbsp) capers (optional)
60 ml (4 tbsp) chopped fresh parsley

Heat the oil in a pan and cook the onion, garlic, shallots and orange rind, if using, for about 5 – 7 minutes until soft. Add the tomatoes and raise the heat until they are cooked to a pulp. Lower the heat, add the fish, stock, water and thyme and bring to a simmer. Cook gently for about 15 minutes, adding the capers for the last 5 minutes. Stir in the parsley or offer separately.

208 Kcal/869 KJ • 34.1 g Protein • 6.3 g Carbohydrate, of which: 5.9 g sugars • 5.3 g Fat, of which: 0.9 g saturates • 0.3 g Sodium • 1.9 g Dietary Fibre

TOM YAM GUNG (HOT AND SOUR SOUP WITH PRAWNS)

450 g (1 lb) raw prawns with shells
900 ml (1½ pints) vegetable stock
2.5 cm (1 inch) piece fresh root ginger, peeled
2 stalks lemon grass, chopped
5 dried red chillies
15 ml (1 tbsp) fish sauce (available from Asian grocers)
5 ml (1 tsp) sugar
1 onion, peeled and chopped into large pieces
100 g (4 oz) button mushrooms, cut into quarters
45 ml (3 tbsp) chopped broad leafed parsley

Peel and devein the prawns. Heat the stock, prawn shells, ginger, lemon grass, chillies, fish sauce, sugar and onion in a saucepan. Bring to the boil and simmer for 20 minutes. Strain through a piece of muslin and return the clear liquid to a large saucepan. Add the mushrooms and prawns to the liquid and cook for 2 minutes. Add parsley, bring to the boil and serve.

64 Kcal/268 KJ • 10.7 g Protein • 3.2 g Carbohydrate, of which: 2.7 g sugars • 1.0 g Fat, of which: 0.1 g saturates • 0.7 g Sodium • 1.1 g Dietary Fibre

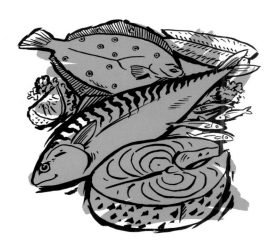

VENISON RAGOUT

750 g (1½ lb) venison, cut into 2.5 cm (1 inch) cubes
25 ml (1 fl oz) red wine vinegar
300 ml (½ pint) good red wine, such as Bordeaux or Rioja
10 whole black peppercorns
4 juniper berries
20 ml (4 tsp) sunflower oil
2 large onions, peeled and chopped
30 ml (2 tbsp) flour
300 ml (½ pint) beef stock
10 ml (2 tsp) redcurrant jelly
100 g (3½ oz) mushrooms, quartered

Combine the venison, vinegar, 100 ml (4 fl oz) of the wine, the peppercorns and juniper berries in a large bowl. Marinate overnight or for at least 4 hours. Drain the venison, reserving the marinade, and pat dry. Heat 10 ml (2 tsp) of the oil in a pan and gently soften the onions for about 8 minutes. Remove the onions from the pan and put into a large flameproof casserole. Add the remaining oil to the pan and brown the venison in batches. Toss each completed batch in flour, then place in the casserole with the onions. When all the venison has been browned, pour the reserved marinade into the pan and bring to the boil. Remove any browned bits from the bottom of the pan. Strain and add to the casserole. Add the remaining wine, the stock and redcurrant jelly and simmer the casserole for 1 hour. Add the mushrooms and cook for at least another 30 minutes or until the meat is tender.

> *376 Kcal/1576 KJ • 40.3 g Protein • 13.6 g Carbohydrate, of which: 6.0 g sugars • 12.7 g Fat, of which: 4.2 g saturates • 0.1 g Sodium • 2.0 g Dietary Fibre*

WEST INDIAN PORK

4 pork loin steaks
1 portion West Indies marinade rub (see page 144)
sunflower oil

Mix together all the ingredients of the West Indies marinade rub. Coat the meat in the mixture and leave for 1 hour. Heat the grill or the barbecue and when hot add the meat. Lightly brush the meat with oil and cook for 5 minutes. Turn the meat over, brush with oil and cook for a further 10 minutes.

> *195 Kcal/812KJ • 23.3 Protein • No Carbohydrate of which no Sugars • 11.2 g Fat, of which: 3.6 g Saturates • 0.1 g Sodium • No Dietary Fibre*

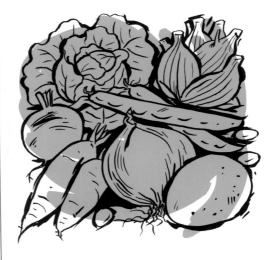

Appendix 1

~ *British Dietary Reference Values* ~

	Percentage of daily total energy/calorie intake		
	Individual minimum	Population average	Individual maximum
Total fat		33 (35)	
Saturated fat		10 (11)	
Polyunsaturates	n – 3 0.2	★6 (6.5)	10
	n – 6 1.0		
Monounsaturates		12 (13)	
★★Trans fatty acids		2 (2)	
Total carbohydrate		47 (50)	
CC foods		37 (39)	
Free sugars	0	10 (11)	
Fibre (non-starch polysaccharides)	12 grams/day	18 g/day	24 g/day

~ *Understanding the table* ~

[*See also WHO table in Chapter Two, page 14*]
The figures in brackets are for those people who do not drink alcohol, which on average accounts for five per cent of food intake. Those who don't drink can eat a little more. Protein is not mentioned, but it accounts for about 15 per cent of calories in Britain. This is much more than is needed but the British experts say it is not necessary to eat less, as it doesn't appear to do any harm at that level.

★ Polyunsaturates are divided into two types: n – 3 (omega – 3) and n – 6 (omega 6). Omega – 3 type can be made in the body from the fatty acids found in oily fish and green leafy vegetables. Omega 6 is found in seeds and plants; the main British dietary sources are sunflower oil, corn oil and the other vegetable oils. Minimum levels have been set to prevent essential fatty acid deficiency. Most of these fatty acids can't be made in the body, and that's why they are called 'essential' fatty acids. For that reason fat cannot be cut out entirely from the diet.

★★ Trans fatty acids. The British line is not to eat more than we currently do – about 5 g ($^1/_4$ oz) a day each, or two per cent of total calories. They are found in cakes, biscuits, vegetable spreads, meat products and milk products. Trans fatty acids develop due to the process of hydrogenation (hardening) of fats to make them more stable and increase shelf-life of foods. Such food processing has led to an increase in trans fatty acid intake. Interest in trans fatty acids has grown because it's been suggested they may be linked to heart disease. However, studies have failed to confirm any link between trans fatty acids and heart disease.

Appendix 2

Dietary Reference Values for vitamin C mg/day

Age	LRNI	EAR	RNI
0–12 mo	6	15	25
1–10 yr	8	20	30
11–14 yr	9	22	35
15+ yr	10	25	40
Additional amounts to be added to pre-pregnancy DRVs			
Pregnant women		+10	
Lactating women		+30	

Dietary Reference Values for vitamin A μg/day retinol equivalent

Age	LRNI		EAR		RNI	
0–12 mo	150		250		350	
1–3 yr	200		300		400	
4–6 yr	200		300		400	
7–10 yr	250		350		500	
11–14 yr	250		400		600	
	Males	Females	Males	Females	Males	Females
15–50+ yr	300	250	500	400	700	600
Additional amounts to be added to pre-pregnancy DRVs						
Pregnant women			+100			
Lactating women			+350			

Dietary Reference Values for thiamin mg/1000 Calories

Thiamin requirements vary according to the number of calories eaten and the amount of exercise taken. The values given are for sedentary lifestyle which applies to most people in the UK.

Age	LRNI	EAR	RNI
0–12 mo	0.20	0.23	0.30
from 1 yr	0.23	0.30	0.40
Examples of DRVs (mg/d)			
Men 19–49 yr	0.60	0.80	1.00
Women 19–49 yr	0.40	0.60	0.80

Dietary Reference Values for riboflavin mg/d

Age	LRNI		EAR		RNI	
0–12 mo	0.2		0.3		0.4	
1–3 yr	0.3		0.5		0.6	
4–6 yr	0.4		0.6		0.8	
7–10 yr	0.5		0.8		1.0	
	Males	Females	Males	Females	Males	Females
11–14 yr	0.8	0.8	1.0	0.9	1.2	1.1
15–18 yr	0.8	0.8	1.0	0.9	1.3	1.1
19–50 yr	0.8	0.8	1.0	0.9	1.3	1.1
Additional amounts to be added to pre-pregnancy DRVs						
Pregnant women			+0.3			
Lactating women			+0.5			

Dietary Reference Values for niacin mg equivalent per 1000 Calories

Niacin requirements vary according to the number of calories eaten and the amount of exercise taken. The values given are for sedentary lifestyle which applies to most people in the UK.

Age	LRNI	EAR	RNI
All ages	4.4	5.5	6.6
Additional amounts to be added to pre-pregnancy DRVs			
Lactating women		+2.3mg/d	
Examples of DRVs (mg/d)			
Men 19–49 yr	11.2	14.0	16.8
Women 19–49 yr	8.5	10.7	12.8

Dietary Reference Values for vitamin B6 mg/g protein

Age	LRNI	EAR	RNI
0–6 mo	3.5	6	8
7–9 mo	6	8	10
10–12 mo	8	10	13
from 1 yr	11	13	15

Examples of DRVs (mg/d) based on actual protein intake (14.7% of total energy) and EARs for energy

		mg/d	
Men 19–49 yr		Energy intake =	2550 Cal
	1.0	1.2	1.4
Women 19–49 yr		Energy intake =	1940 Cal
	0.8	0.9	1.2

Dietary Reference Values for vitamin B12 µg/day

Age	LRNI	EAR	RNI
0–6 mo	0.10	0.25	0.30
7–12 mo	0.25	0.35	0.40
1–3 yr	0.30	0.40	0.50
4–6 yr	0.50	0.70	0.80
7–10 yr	0.60	0.80	1.00
11–14 yr	0.80	1.00	1.20
15+ yr	1.00	1.25	1.50
Additional amounts to be added to pre-pregnancy DRVs			
Lactating women		+0.5	

Dietary Reference Values for folate µg/day

Age	LRNI	EAR	RNI
0–12 mo	30	40	50
1–3 yr	35	50	70
4–6 yr	50	75	100
7–10 yr	75	110	150
11+ yr	100	150	200
Additional amounts to be added to pre-pregnancy DRVs			
Pregnant women		+100	
Lactating women		+60	

Dietary Reference Values for vitamin D µg/day

Age	RNI	
0–up to 6 mo	8.5	
6 mo–3 yr	7.0	
4–64 yr	0	provided skin is exposed to sun
65+ yr	10.0	
Pregnant and Lactating women	10.0	

Dietary Reference Values for calcium mg/d

Age	LRNI		EAR		RNI	
0–12 mo	240		400		525	
1–3 yr	200		275		350	
4–6 yr	275		350		450	
7–10 yr	325		425		550	
	Males	Females	Males	Females	Males	Females
11–14 yr	450	480	750	625	1,000	800
15–18 yr	450	480	750	625	1,000	800
19+ yr	400	400	525	525	700	700
Additional amounts to be added to pre-pregnancy DRVs						
Lactating women			+550			

Dietary Reference Values for iron mg/day

Age	LRNI		EAR		RNI	
0–3 mo	0.9		1.3		1.7	
4–6 mo	2.3		3.3		4.3	
7–12 mo	4.2		6.0		7.8	
1–3 yr	3.7		5.3		6.9	
4–6 yr	3.3		4.7		6.1	
7–10 yr	4.7		6.7		8.7	
	Males	Females	Males	Females	Males	Females
11–18 yr	6.1	8.0★	8.7	11.4★	11.3	14.8★
19–49 yr	4.7	8.0★	6.7	11.4★	8.7	14.8★
50+ yr	4.7	4.7	6.7	6.7	8.7	8.7

★ About 10% of women with very high menstrual losses will need more iron than shown. Their needs are best met by taking iron supplements.

Dietary Reference Values for zinc mg/day

Age	LRNI		EAR		RNI	
0–6 mo	2.6		3.3		4.0	
7 mo–3 yr	3.0		3.8		5.0	
4–6 yr	4.0		5.0		6.5	
7–10 yr	4.0		5.4		7.0	
11–14 yr	5.3		7.0		9.0	
	Males	Females	Males	Females	Males	Females
15+ yr	5.5	4.0	7.3	5.5	9.5	7.0
Additional amounts to be added to pre-pregnancy DRVs						
Lactating women	0–4 mo		+6.0			
	4+ mo		+2.5			

Dietary Reference Values for potassium mg/d

Age	LRNI	RNI
0–3 mo	400	800
4–6 mo	400	850
7–9 mo	400	700
10–12 mo	450	700
1–3 yr	450	800
4–6 yr	600	1100
7–10 yr	950	2000
11–14 y	1600	3100
15+ yr	2000	3500

Dietary Reference Values for selenium µg/day

Age	LRNI	RNI		
0–3 mo	4	10		
4–6 mo	5	13		
7–9 mo	5	10		
10–12 mo	6	10		
1–3 yr	7	15		
4–6 yr	10	20		
7–10 yr	16	30		
11–14 yr	25	45		
	Males	Females	Males	Females
15–18 yr	40	40	70	60
19+ yr	40	40	75	60
Lactating women	+15		+15	

Dietary Reference Values for sodium mg/day

Age	LRNI	RNI
0–3 mo	140	210
4–6 mo	140	280
7–9 mo	200	320
10–12 mo	200	350
1–3 yr	200	500
4–6 yr	280	700
7–10 yr	350	1200
11–14 yr	460	1600
15+ yr	575	1600

Appendix 3

Estimated Average Requirements (EARs) for Energy

Age	EARs MJ/day (Cal/day)			
	males		females	
0–3 mo	2.28	(545)	2.16	(515)
4–6 mo	2.89	(690)	2.69	(645)
7–9 mo	3.44	(825)	3.20	(765)
10–12 mo	3.85	(920)	3.61	(865)
1–3 yr	5.15	(1,230)	4.86	(1,165)
4–6 yr	7.16	(1,715)	6.46	(1,545)
7–10 yr	8.24	(1,970)	7.28	(1,740)
11–14 yr	9.27	(2,220)	7.92	(1,845)
15–18 yr	11.51	(2,755)	8.83	(2,110)
19–50 yr	10.60	(2,550)	8.10	(1,940)
51–59 yr	10.60	(2,550)	8.00	(1,900)
60–64 yr	9.93	(2,380)	7.99	(1,900)
65–74 yr	9.71	(2,330)	7.96	(1,900)
75+ years	8.77	(2,100)	7.61	(1,810)
Pregnancy			+0.80 •	(200)
Lactation:				
1 month			+1.90	(450)
2 months			+2.20	(530)
3 months			+2.40	(570)
4–6 months (Group 1)			+2.00	(480)
4–6 months (Group 2)			+2.40	(570)
> 6 months (Group 1)			+1.00	(240)
> 6 months (Group 2)			+2.30	(550)

•Last trimester only

~ Index ~